THEORY-DIRECTED NURSING PRACTICE

Shirley Melat Ziegler, PhD, RN, is a Professor in the College of Nursing, Texas Woman's University. She teaches Practice Oriented Nursing Theory and Collaborative Nursing Practice in the masters' program. She received a BSNEd in psychiatric-mental health nursing from the University of Pittsburgh, an MA in psychiatric-mental health nursing from New York University, and a PhD in nursing from the University of Texas at Austin. She is the senior author of the text *Nursing Diagnosis, Nursing Process, and Nursing Knowledge: Avenues to Autonomy.*

THEORY-DIRECTED NURSING PRACTICE

Shirley M. Ziegler, PhD, RN
Editor

SPRINGER PUBLISHING COMPANY
NEW YORK

Springer Publishing Company, Inc
536 Broadway
New York, NY 10012-3955

93 94 95 96 97 / 5 4 3 2 1

Library of Congress Cataloging-in-Publication Data

Theory-directed nursing practice / Shirley Melat Ziegler, editor.
    p. cm.
    Includes bibliographical references and index.
    ISBN 0-8261-7630-5
    1. Nursing. 2. Nursing—Philosophy. I. Ziegler, Shirley Melat.
    [DNLM: 1. Nursing Care—methods. 2. Nursing Theory. WY 100
    T396]
    RT42.T44 1993
    610.73'01—dc20
    DNLM/DLC
    for Library of Congress   92-2379
                                                CIP

This book is dedicated to the graduate faculty and graduate students of the College of Nursing, Texas Woman's University, Dallas Center. They have worked diligently to describe and implement a strategy for using scientific theory in nursing practice.

Contents

Contributors

Wilda K. Arnold, EdD, RN, is an Associate Professor in the College of Nursing at Texas Woman's University. She teaches both undergraduate and graduate psychiatric-mental health nursing and group dynamics. She earned her BS in nursing from Northwestern State University, MS in nursing from Texas Woman's University, and an EdD in secondary and higher education from East Texas State University. She is a member of a number of organizations.

Kathleen M. Baldwin, PHD, RN, CEN, CCRN, is an Assistant Professor in the College of Nursing at Texas Woman's University. She teaches undergraduate medical-surgical nursing. She is a graduate of the Western Pennsylvania Hospital School of Nursing. She holds BS, MS, and PhD degrees in nursing from Texas Woman's University. She is certified in emergency nursing and critical care nursing.

Susan Goad, EdD, RN, is a Professor in the College of Nursing at Texas Woman's University. She teaches medical surgical nursing and nursing administration at the graduate level. She earned her BS in nursing from Incarnate Word, MS in nursing from Texas Woman's University, and an EdD from the University of Houston.

Lois Hough, PhD, RN, is Assistant Dean of Nursing at the Dallas Center of Texas Woman's University. She teaches medical surgical nursing and clinical nurse specialist role at the graduate level. She earned a BS from Florida State University, an MS from University of California, and a PhD from Walden University.

Oneida M. Hughes, PhD, RN, is a Professor in the College of Nursing at Texas Woman's University. She teaches medical-surgical nursing, nursing ethics, and nurse educator role in the graduate program. She holds a BS from the University of Texas at Galveston, an MSN from Indiana University School of Nursing, and a PhD in higher education from North Texas State University. She is a member of American Nurses' Association and Sigma Theta Tau.

Judy Johnson-Russell, EdD, RN, is an Assistant Professor in the College of Nursing at Texas Woman's University. She has taught pediatrics and nurse practitioner courses for over 20 years. She holds a BSN degree from the University of Arkansas, an MS in Nursing from Boston University, and an EdD in Marriage and Family Counseling from East Texas State University. She is a member of Sigma Theta Tau, American Association of Counseling and Development, Texas Association of Counseling and Development, and the American Association of Marriage and Family Therapists.

Terry L. Jones, MS, RN, CCRN, is the coordinator of critical care nursing education at Parkland Memorial Hospital. She has worked in critical care in the roles of staff nurse, assistant head nurse, and nurse educator. She completed her CCRN certification and is active in the American Association of Critical Care Nurses. She received her BSN from Marycrest College in Davenport, Iowa and her MS from Texas Woman's University.

Caryl Erhardt Mobley, PHD, RN, is an Assistant Professor in the College of Nursing at Texas Woman's University. She teaches maternal–child health nursing in both the undergraduate and graduate program. She received her BSN from Duke University, her MSN in maternal–child health from the University of North Carolina at Chapel Hill, and her PhD in Human Development and Communication Sciences from the University of Texas at Dallas. Dr. Mobley is a vice president of Beta Beta Chapter of Sigma Theta Tau and a member of the Society for Research in Child Development.

Rose M. Nieswiadomy, PhD, RN, is a Professor in the College of Nursing at Texas Woman's University. She is the coordinator of the nursing' master's program at the Dallas Center of Texas Woman's University and teaches both undergraduate and graduate nursing research. She received a BS and an MS in nursing from Texas Woman's University and a PhD in higher education from North Texas State University. She is on the Board of Directors of District 4, Texas Nurses' Association. She is a member of ANA, NLN, Sigma Theta Tau, the Council of Nurse Researchers, Southern Research Society, and the American Nurses' Foundation Century Club. She is the author of the textbook, *Foundations of Nursing Research*.

Gail Walden Watson, EdD, RN, is an Associate Professor in the College of Nursing at Texas Woman's University. She teaches maternal–child health at the graduate level and undergraduate nursing assessment. She holds a BS from Texas Woman's University, an MS from Boston University, and an EdD from East Texas State University. She is a member of the American Nurses' Association and Sigma Theta Tau. She serves as President of the Dallas Chapter of the Vietnam Veterans of America, Inc.

Preface

Nursing is becoming an autonomous profession with a unique body of knowledge. At the least there is an adapted body of knowledge that is pertinent to nursing. For many years nurses have based nursing care on insufficient methods of knowing, such as intuition and trial and error. Nurses need a better source of knowledge, information that describes: "If the nurse does X, Y will happen, and the reason it will happen is because. . . ." This can be achieved by presenting a composite of selected theories that lend themselves to application in nursing practice. This book illustrates the use of theory to guide, plan, implement, and evaluate nursing practice.

The book provides a sampling of theories deemed relevant to nursing. Nine Chapters discuss the application of a specific theory to a specific clinical situation. The final chapter describes a general nursing strategy for the nurse to use in linking scientific theory with practice. It is hoped that this book will assist nurses interested in strengthening their practice by the use of theory, especially psychosocial theory.

In the complex world of nursing, theories from various scientific fields can be applied. Biology, chemistry, medical science, psychology, and, of course, nursing science itself all can contribute theoretical insights to nursing practice. In this book, well-known theories, primarily psychosocial, were explored as to their applicability to the work of nurses. A widely accepted definition of nursing is "the diagnosis and treatment of human responses to actual or potential health problems" (American Nurses' Association, 1980, p. 9). Therefore, nurses need to develop competence in observing, evaluating, and influencing human behavior. This competence has, of course, grown in many nurses through observation and intuition. With this book the link between outstanding theorists and the professional work of nurses is firmly established.

References

American Nurses' Association. (1980). *Nursing: A social policy statement*. Kansas City, MO: Author.

Chapter 1

Introduction to Theory-Directed Nursing Practice

Shirley Melat Ziegler

The nurse in practice may be seen as the link between scientific theory and the delivery of quality nursing care—that is, between knowledge and action. In what way does the nurse in practice think? How does the way the nurse thinks affect the delivery of nursing care? These are critical questions and the way these questions are answered is also critical. It influences (1) the quality of nursing care delivered, (2) how students are taught, (3) the research designed to test theory, and (4) the type of theory to be generated and developed. If the nurse in practice does not function as this vital link, there is no link between what is known and what is practiced; the dichotomy between theory and practice will continue.

Scientific theory and nursing practice have different purposes. The purpose of scientific theory in nursing is to describe, explain, predict, and give a sense of understanding of some phenomenon deemed relevant to nurses. The purpose of nursing practice is to use the understanding provided by scientific theory to bring about a change in the health responses of clients or a change in health care settings. However, theory does not lead directly to practice. Nor does practice lead directly to theory. A strategy to apply theory to practice is required.

The proposed strategy is based on the following assumptions:

- Rarely do nurses face a nursing situation that consists of a single problem. Rather, nurses face many problems on many levels.
- Problems have more than a single solution.
- Clinical decisions are difficult and outcomes are uncertain.
- Nurses are constantly making choices. These choices are often based on too little knowledge and involve guessing (hypothesizing) about the outcomes of nursing actions. These guesses are most valid if based on theory that has been supported by research.
- Nursing actions, even if based on theory, are still creative acts.

THEORY-DIRECTED NURSING PRACTICE

Theory-directed nursing practice begins in the world of practice; it begins with a practice that needs to be considered. Faced with a clinical situation, the nurse begins to describe, explain, and predict an aspect of nursing reality by addressing the following questions:

1. What conditions exist in the situation?
2. What conditions in the situation need to be changed?
3. What theory or theories address the conditions that need to be changed?
4. Which of the predictive/explanatory theories will be used to guide actions in this practice situation?
5. What are the concepts of the theory?
6. What are the definitions and empirical indicators of these concepts?
7. What situational variables need to be assessed that are pertinent to the concepts of the theory and the conditions that need to be changed?
8. How do the theory's relational statements identify and explain those variables (risk factors) that, if present, could be used to predict the possibility of a future condition needing to be changed (primary prevention)?
9. How do the theory's relational statements identify and explain the causes of the conditions that need to be changed?
10. What are the causes of the conditions needing change that are amenable to nursing manipulation?
11. What are the norms for the events described in the theory that could

be used as standards for comparing client or situational data characteristics?

12. What are the "model" nursing diagnoses or situational problems suggested by this theory?

13. What are the interventions that can be planned and that can be expected to modify the causative variables?

The nurse observes a discrepancy between the way events are and the way events should be. A discrepancy may be directly observed or observed and reported by others. Faced with a discrepancy, the nurse uses the reasoning process of induction in seeking answers to the following questions:

- Of what patterns are these observations a part?
- What problems do these patterns infer?
- Who has the problem?
- What are the theories that address these problematic patterns?

The nurse links the data observed in practice to the theories she or he remembers. Each theory presents suggestions as to the probable cause of the observed data considered problematic. As the etiological explanation varies, so do the implications for intervention. The nurse needs to decide which of the theories will be used to guide interventions in the practice situation.

Few guidelines exist for the selection of theory in a given practice situation. A nurse must have prior knowledge of existing theories in order to select an appropriate one for a specific situation. A nurse must link some observation in the practice situation to a pattern described in the theory (diagnostic reasoning). When a situation in practice is seen as problematic, the nurse locates a theory, or a portion of a theory, which is perceived as appropriate to the problem situation. The reasoning process of deduction is used in moving back from the theory to the events observed in the practice situation.

The nurse validates hunches regarding the link between a theory and the situation by conducting additional observations of the events in practice. This assessment is theory-driven by the use of hypothesis(es). The nurse reasons that if a theory is relevant to the situation, certain additional patterns should be identifiable. If the patterns predicted by the theory are found, the nurse develops a strategy to deal with the problem based on the theory. If the patterns predicted by the theory are not found, additional hypotheses deduced from other theories are generated until a match is found.

FORMAT OF THEORY APPLICATION CHAPTERS

The format for each chapter in this book is the same. A clinical case vignette
is presented first because nursing problems begin in practice. Possible theories that address the patterns in the practice situation are proposed. The
various causes for the patterns predicted by the theories are contrasted. One
of the theories is then selected for application and the chosen theory is
discussed. Its major concepts are identified, a clinical example of each of the
concepts is given, and these concepts are linked into the major relational
statements. Phenomena encompassed by the theory, viewed as problematic
to nurses, are identified, including the causes. Model nursing diagnoses or
situational problems suggested by the theory are listed and nursing interventions derived from the theory are identified. Finally, a diagnosis-
directed nursing care plan or a plan for nursing action is presented for the
case and supported with the propositional statements from the theory. For
those readers wishing more information regarding the theories briefly introduced as applicable, recommended readings appear at the end of each
chapter.

Chapter 2

Aguilera and Messick's Theory of Crisis Intervention

Terry L. Jones

The presence of an acute life threatening illness in one family member may throw the family system into turmoil. The added stressors associated with a critical illness challenge the family's coping resources and problem-solving abilities on several levels. Nurses caring for critically ill patients and their families frequently assist family members in their struggle to cope with such stressors and to maintain system integrity (Hodovanic, Reardon, Reese, & Hedges, 1984). The case of Mary Brown and her family will illustrate how the nurse can use Aguilera and Messick's theory of crisis intervention to assist families in their struggle to cope effectively.

The Brown case will be presented followed by a summary of three theories that could potentially be used to direct the nursing care for this family. One of these theories, Aguilera and Messick's theory of crisis intervention, will be discussed in greater depth. A demonstration of how the theory of crisis intervention can be used to guide the nursing care for the Brown family will be provided.

CLIENT CASE

Mary Brown is a 25-year-old white female who is approximately 25 weeks pregnant. She presented to the OB clinic with a 5-day history of cold and

5

flu-like symptoms, including a persistent cough. At this time she was found to be dyspneic with a respiratory rate of 28 and mildly diaphoretic. Physical exam revealed coarse rales and ronchi throughout all lung fields, sinus tachycardia, and an oral temperature of 39.5°C. A chest x-ray revealed bilateral pulmonary infiltrates and other laboratory data showed mild hypoxemia with hypocapnea, and a WBC of 20.9. Her social history was significant for a 3-year-old son recovering from chicken pox and no history of drug or alcohol abuse.

A tentative diagnosis of varicella pneumonia was made and Mary was admitted to the Medical Intensive Care Unit (MICU) and placed on respiratory isolation. Upon admission, external uterine and fetal heart monitors were placed revealing fetal tachycardia but no uterine activity. Pelvic exam revealed a closed cervix and intact membranes. Mary's treatment consisted of administration of oxygen via 40% Venturi mask, broad spectrum antibiotics, antipyretics, maintenance IV fluids via peripheral veins, and placement of an arterial line for hemodynamic monitoring and frequent phlebotomy. Over the next 2 days Mary's dyspnea worsened despite oxygenation with a 100% nonrebreathing mask. She became increasingly lethargic and her arterial blood gases revealed profound hypoxemia and respiratory acidosis.

Mary was subsequently orally intubated and mechanical ventilation initiated. Despite mechanical ventilation, however, mild hypoxemia persisted and based on her chest x-ray, as well as physical and laboratory exam, a diagnosis of adult respiratory distress syndrome (ARDS) and sepsis secondary to varicella pneumonia was made. Heavy sedation and neuromuscular blockade were instituted to facilitate effective ventilation and a thermodilution catheter was inserted to monitor her hemodynamic status. By midday the nurse noted that Mary was having mild contractions. Conventional methods to suppress labor were contraindicated due to ARDS; thus, her labor was allowed to continue despite the concomitant poor prognosis for the fetus and potential adverse effects for Mary.

During visiting hours the nurse caring for Mary, Ms. Johnson, observed that Mary's husband was reluctant to enter her room. Mr. Brown stood outside her door sobbing as he stared through her window. Ms. Johnson provided an isolation gown and mask and encouraged Mr. Brown to enter the room. Once at the bedside Mr. Brown continued to sob even louder than before and did not attempt to touch his wife. The only words he spoke were, "I'm sorry Mary. Please don't die." When asked if he had any questions for the medical or nursing staff, Mr. Brown shook his head "no" and left, never making eye contact.

Later in the day Mary's sisters appeared during visiting hours. Ms. Johnson observed that they directed several questions to the nursing staff regarding Mary's condition as well as the sequence of events leading to her admission, but did not speak to Mr. Brown. When Mr. Brown's parents arrived shortly thereafter, the nurse witnessed a few heated exchanges between them and Mary's sisters. Ms. Johnson scheduled a family conference to provide a progress report on Mary's condition. During the conference she noticed that Mr. Brown asked no questions, made no comments, and made eye contact with no one. After the conference Ms. Johnson spoke with Mr. Brown's parents. They informed her that their son had not been home to sleep or to see his son since Mary's admission. "He just doesn't know what to do. He is so worried that Mary is going to die; he blames himself for not getting her to the doctor sooner." When questioned about Mr. Brown's apparent withdrawal, they reported that, "Whenever he's troubled about something, he just gets that way. He doesn't ever say much—just keeps to himself. When he was a kid he would just go to his room or somewhere else to be by himself—kind of like he just wanted to think things through." They further reported that Mr. Brown had not experienced the death of a close friend or family member before. Mr. Brown's parents appeared genuinely concerned for their son and were open in their display of affection.

PATTERNING CUES FROM THE CLIENT CASE

The nurse recognizes that an acute life-threatening illness such as Mary's can inflict a tremendous amount of stress on family members. Based on her knowledge of responses to stressors, the nurse concludes that Mr. Brown is experiencing an unhealthful response to Mary's illness. More specifically, she determines that the patterns of behavior exhibited by the Brown family are not resulting in a sense of control of the situation. Ms. Johnson identifies the following cues:

Mary and her unborn child are in critical condition.
Mr. Brown fears the death of his wife and/or his unborn child.
Mr. Brown has withdrawn from social interaction.
Mr. Brown has neglected his normal daily activities.
Mr. Brown has begun to neglect his basic needs.

By organizing these cues into a pattern, Ms. Johnson realizes that prompt intervention must be instituted to help Mr. Brown change his behavior pattern reflecting severe emotional distress to a behavior pattern reflecting his usual emotional state. Ms. Johnson must first identify the factors that precipitated such a severe state of tension and then determine how to nullify their effects. She must begin this step by linking the pattern of cues from the Brown case to her knowledge of pertinent theories.

SELECTED RELEVANT THEORIES

A variety of theories could be used to direct the care for the Brown family. Three such theories will be presented in this chapter to illustrate how various theoretical approaches can result in different explanations for behavior and thus call for different nursing interventions. The theories presented here are coping (Lazarus & Folkman, 1984), grief (Lindemann, 1944), and crisis intervention (Aguilera, 1990; Aguilera & Messick, 1986).

Lazarus and Folkman's Theory of Coping

One theory that might be considered for this case is the coping process described by Lazarus and Folkman (1984). They define coping as, ". . . constantly changing cognitive and behavioral efforts to manage specific external and/or internal demands that are appraised as taxing or exceeding the resources of the person" (p. 141). The process of coping serves two major purposes—managing the problem and regulating the emotions elicited by the problem. The steps involved in coping are those of primary appraisal, secondary appraisal, and reappraisal. These steps involve the individual making judgements with regard to the degree of threat posed by the stressor as well as the resources available to manage the stressor.

The behavior selected to manage the problem and its associated emotions depends on the results of the appraisal process and available resources. Such behavior is effective to the extent that it fulfills both purposes; the problem is managed without great emotional cost. Major causes of ineffective coping have been identified as inaccurate appraisal (primary or secondary) and inadequate coping resources. Interventions would involve assisting the client in achieving accurate appraisal of the event and helping the client access coping resources.

The nursing diagnosis generated for Mr. Brown from this theory is "emotional distress related to inadequate coping resources." Nursing interventions for Mr. Brown would be directed at helping him access coping resources not previously utilized by him.

Lindemann's Grief Theory

Another theory that might be considered for the Brown case is that of grief as described by Lindemann (1944). According to Lindemann, persons experiencing acute grief display a syndrome of common behaviors. Such behaviors are classified into the categories of somatic distress, preoccupation with the image of the deceased, guilt, hostile reactions, and loss of patterns of conduct. Lindemann suggests that such behaviors are also resolved through a common process known as "grief work." This grief work involves, "emancipation from bondage to the deceased, readjustment to the environment in which the deceased is missing, and the formation of new relationships" (p. 143). Failure to complete this process may result in distorted grief reactions.

Lindemann further contends that in addition to actual death, such grief reactions can be precipitated by a loss due to a separation or to a threat of separation or threat of death. When in response to the threat of separation or death, such behaviors are termed anticipatory grief reactions.

The nursing diagnosis generated for the Brown case from this theory is "emotional distress related to inadequate anticipatory grief work." Nursing interventions would focus on assisting the client through the anticipatory grief process.

Aguilera and Messick's Theory of Crisis Intervention

Aguilera and Messick's theory of crisis intervention considers how a state of psychological disequilibrium is precipitated as well as the mechanisms through which equilibrium is regained or crisis evolves. The state of psychological equilibrium is seen as being continuously threatened by stressors. Through a problem-solving process and effective utilization of coping skills, equilibrium can be maintained. Should the usual methods of problem solving and coping be insufficient to handle a stressor, a state of severe disequilibrium may occur, accompanied by unhealthful behavioral responses. Because

Aguilera and Messick's theory of crisis intervention offers an explanation of the unhealthful behavior exhibited by Mr. Brown and provides guidelines for facilitating effective problem solving in the context of an acute setting, it has been selected for illustration in this client situation.

DESCRIPTION OF AGUILERA AND MESSICK'S THEORY OF CRISIS INTERVENTION

Aguilera and Messick first described their theory of crisis intervention in 1970 and have since produced a number of updated editions of the original publication (1974, 1978, 1982, and 1986). The most recent edition, however, has been revised by Aguilera alone. The description of crisis intervention here is taken from Aguilera's 1990 publication, which has not greatly deviated from the earlier editions. Thus, the theory will be referred to as Aguilera and Messick's.

Although the focus of this chapter is on the paradigm of intervention developed by Aguilera and Messick, it must be pointed out that the foundation of crisis theory was generated by Caplan (1964). It was Caplan who suggested that in the quest to maintain equilibrium individuals are constantly called on to solve problems. As long as individuals perceive that the problems faced can be solved using their available coping skills, equilibrium is maintained. The perception that a problem cannot be readily solved using previously effective coping skills will result in a rise in tension and sense of disequilibrium. A crisis is precipitated at this point unless alternatives can be found. The perception that one will be unable to find an acceptable solution to the problem will result in feelings of anxiety, fear, guilt, shame, and helplessness. The behavioral responses to such feelings, whether consciously or unconsciously activated, can be unhealthful. For a more detailed discussion of the development of a crisis the reader is encouraged to consult Caplan's original work (1964).

Major Concepts

There are basically three factors that work together to determine whether or not a crisis, and thus unhealthful behavior, will evolve after a crisis-precipitating event. These factors are referred to as balancing factors and, when intact, function to restore equilibrium. The balancing factors (perception of the event, situational support, and available coping mechanisms), along with the crisis and the crisis-precipitating event, are the major concepts of the theory and will be named and defined. Table 2.1 presents a summary of these major concepts and subconcepts.

Table 2.1   Selected Concepts of Aguilera and Messick's Theory of Crisis Intervention

Crisis
Crisis-Precipitating Event
   Situational Crisis
   Maturational Crisis
Balancing Factors
   Perception of the Event
     Primary Appraisal
     Secondary Appraisal
     Reappraisal
   Available Support Systems
   Available Coping Mechanisms

Theoretical Definitions of Major Concepts

Crisis

According to Aguilera (1990) when faced with day-to-day problems, equilibrium is maintained to the extent that customary problem-solving techniques are effective. When such problems cannot be readily solved with customary techniques, the result is a state of crisis in which, "there is a rise in inner tension, there are signs of anxiety, and there is disorganization of function resulting in a protracted period of emotional upset" (p. 5). Crisis is characterized by a feeling of helplessness to the point where the individual is unable to take an active role in solving the problem.

Crisis-Precipitating Event

Crisis-precipitating event refers to stressful events that could precipitate a crisis. Aguilera and Messick have identified two types, situational and maturational. A Situational Crisis is the result of crisis-precipitating events such as the birth of a premature infant, divorce, rape, or death of a loved one. Maturational Crisis refers to potential crisis areas occurring "during the periods of great social, physical, and psychological change experienced by all human beings in the normal growth process" (p. 204).

Balancing Factors

Balancing factors are variables that exist between the individual's perception of disequilibrium and the resolution of the problem. The three balancing factors are perception of the event, situational support, and available coping mechanisms.

1. *Perception of the Event* refers to the "cognition or subjective meaning" an individual places on events (Aguilera, 1990, p. 68). The process of creating one's perception of events in turn involves the concept of *appraisal*. The process of appraisal is "the ongoing perceptual process by which a potentially harmful event is distinguished from a potentially benign or irrelevant event in one's life" (p. 68).
   a. *primary appraisal* refers to the process of making a judgement in regard to "the perceived outcome of the event in relation to one's future goals and values" (p. 68).
   b. *secondary appraisal* refers to the process "whereby one perceives the range of coping alternatives available either to master the threat or to achieve a beneficial outcome" (p. 68).
   c. *reappraisal* refers to "changes in the original perception as a result of changes in the environment" (p. 68).
2. *Available Situational Support* refers to "those persons who are available in the environment and who can be depended on to help solve the problem" (p. 70).
3. *Coping Mechanisms* refer to behaviors aimed at reducing the psychological tension associated with a perceived threat to psychological equilibrium. These behaviors may be consciously or unconsciously employed. *Available coping mechanisms* refer to those behaviors that have been "used at some time in the developmental past of the individual and been found effective in maintaining emotional stability, and have become part of his lifestyle in meeting and dealing with the stressors of daily living" (p. 73).

Examples of Concepts Relevant to Clinical Practice

Clinical examples of the major concepts are as follows.

Crisis-Precipitating Event

A mother is notified that her 18-year-old son has been admitted to the intensive care unit following a high speed motor vehicle accident in which he suffered multiple injuries (situational crisis).

Perception of the Event

Upon receiving this information she recalls that her father died in an intensive care unit less than 6 months ago and that her best friend's husband died as a result of a motor vehicle accident several years ago. Based on her previous experiences and current knowledge of the event, this mother identifies this situation as being a serious emergency that might well result in devastating consequences (primary appraisal). Fearing that her son might die, she leaves work immediately and rushes to the hospital to be with her son. At this point in time she doesn't know what else to do but wait and pray (secondary appraisal). Later that evening the physician informs her that although alive and in no immediate danger of dying, her son's injuries would likely leave him paralyzed from the waist down. With the fear of her son's death subsiding, this mother's thoughts now center on how her son will react to the paralysis (reappraisal).

Situational Support

Frightened by the news of her son's injuries and in anticipation of the many problems and decisions that lay ahead, this mother, now joined by her husband, calls her family and friends to be with her. She arranges for her neighbors to transport out-of-town grandparents from the airport. Her best friend will stay with her at the hospital while her husband is at work, and the ladies' club at the church will provide meals for the younger children at home. Her sister will get the children off to school in the morning and pick them up in the afternoon.

Coping Mechanisms

As with past problems this mother responds by attempting to gain control of the situation. She demands daily conferences with her son's caregivers in an attempt to maintain an understanding of his condition and to ensure herself an active role in the decisions made regarding his care. In addition she visits the chapel every day and insists that the minister from her church visit her son at least three times a week. She also arranges for some of her son's friends to visit during the afternoon and evening visiting hours every day to keep his spirits up.

Crisis

Despite her attempt to solve the problem using customary problem-solving techniques (attempting to control the situation) this mother begins to display signs of emotional disequilibrium. She remains at the hospital 24 hours a day, sleeps only during brief intervals, and reports having no appetite. When she receives a notice that her sick leave at work has expired, this mother begins to cry hysterically and states, "I just can't handle any more of this. What am I going to do?"

Major Relational Statements

The relational statements which serve to link the major concepts are presented. Aguilera and Messick suggest that the status of psychological equilibrium is directly related to the status of balancing factors, that is, perception of the event, situational support, and available coping mechanisms. If all of the balancing factors are intact, the problem will be resolved, equilibrium regained, and a crisis avoided. If, on the other hand, there is a weakness in any one or more of the balancing factors, then resolution of the problem will not occur, the disequilibrium continues, and a crisis is precipitated.

The perception of the event is said to be intact to the extent that it is a realistic perception. A distorted perception of the event, or of one's ability to cope with the event, will result in ineffective problem solving and thus an increase in psychological tension. Situational supports are said to be intact to the extent that they provide positive feedback in regard to one's self-worth and problem-solving ability. Failure to receive such support, whether actual or perceived, can disrupt one's sense of psychological equilibrium and thus precipitate a crisis. Aguilera and Messick further suggest that one's need to seek situational support increases as the perceived threat increases and the self-esteem decreases.

Coping mechanisms are said to be adequate to the extent that they are effective in reducing psychological tension and do not interfere with the activities of daily living. Aguilera and Messick suggest that individuals tend to respond to a stressor with coping mechanisms that have been successful in reducing the psychological tension in similar situations in the past. Over a period of time such responses are essentially activated on an unconscious level at the onset of the stressor such that one experiences minimal psychological discomfort. Should those usual responses be ineffective against the stressor, the discomfort becomes conscious followed by psychological disequilibrium and crisis.

IMPLICATIONS OF AGUILERA AND MESSICK'S THEORY OF CRISIS INTERVENTION FOR CLINICAL PRACTICE

This section presents the use of Aguilera and Messick's theory in nursing practice. Factors to be assessed, methods of assessing, theory-specific diagnoses, care planning, and evaluation of care are discussed.

Factors to be Assessed and Methods of Assessing

An initial assessment is made to ascertain whether or not a crisis situation exists. Through direct questioning and observation, information regarding the presence and extent of emotional tension experienced by the client is obtained. The focus is on the client's level of functioning with respect to problem-solving ability. A determination is made as to whether or not a state of emotional tension exists and whether or not the client is presently capable of participating in effective problem solving.

Because a crisis is generally thought of as being self-limited, the focus is on the immediate problem and, therefore, a detailed description of the client's past history is not a priority. The crisis event typically occurs within 10 to 14 days of the time help is sought (Aguilera, 1990). An assessment is made regarding the client's perception of the crisis event. This information is gained through direct questioning as well as observation. The goal is to define the problem and precipitating events as specifically as possible. An assessment is also made at this time as to what barriers exist to problem solving.

The balancing factors are also assessed. Once the crisis is identified, an assessment is made as to what meaning the event has to the client in terms of his or her value system and future plans. A determination is then made as to the extent of congruency between the client's perception of the event and the reality of the situation. An assessment is also made as to whether or not the client recognizes the relationship between the event described and the perceived stress. And finally, an assessment is made as to what the client perceives as alternatives in the problem-solving process.

In the assessment of the client's available situational supports, the client's perception is once again a point of focus. Individuals are identified whom the client perceives as supportive, trustworthy, and available and willing to help. Again, this information is gained through direct questioning and observation.

Finally, the assessment of available coping skills is made. The focus here is on what the client usually does when faced with a problem that is difficult to solve. Whether or not such usual coping methods have been tried is assessed as well as whether or not a similar problem has been encountered. The client's perception of the effectiveness of his or her coping skills is assessed as well as perceptions of what might work in the future.

It is also important to determine if the client is at risk for suicide or homicide. If a risk for either exists, then making appropriate arrangements must become the priority.

Theory Specific Diagnoses

Sample nursing diagnoses are presented that are specific to Aguilera and Messick's theory of crisis intervention. They focus on the balancing factors that influence effective problem solving.

Response

Aguilera and Messick's theory of crisis intervention is helpful in generating the response component of theory-specific nursing diagnoses. The response component of the nursing diagnosis statement is crisis. Examples of behaviors that may be considered defining characteristics of crisis are: anxiety, anger, hostility, withdrawal, perceived powerlessness, perceived helplessness, hopelessness, fear, feelings of failure, low self-esteem, self-destructive behavior, and lack of participation in decision making.

Etiology

Etiology components for the nursing diagnosis statements could reflect weaknesses in any of the balancing factors. Examples of etiologies that reflect weaknesses in the perception of the event include:

- The client's perception of the event may be distorted from reality.
- The client may not understand the relationship between the event and feelings of tension.
- The client may perceive that the problem is unsolvable.

Examples of etiologies that reflect weaknesses in available situational support include:

- The client may have a lack of knowledge of how to access community and institutional support systems.
- The client may be geographically separated from identified support persons.
- The client may perceive that he or she has no available support.
- The client's perceived support persons may not be equipped to provide the kind of support needed for the problem at hand.

Examples of etiologies that reflect weaknesses in the available coping mechanisms include:

- The client's usual coping mechanisms have been ineffective.
- The client has not activated all of his or her usual coping mechanisms in attempt to solve the problem.

● The client has failed to identify new coping skills in attempt to solve the problem.

Sample Nursing Diagnoses

A selection from the response and etiology examples generated from Aguilera and Messick's theory of crisis intervention was used to generate the following nursing diagnoses.

Crisis related to failure to understand the relationship between the event and feelings of tension. "If the perception of the event is distorted, a relationship between the event and feelings of stress may not be recognized. Thus, attempts to solve the problem will be ineffective, and tension will not be reduced" (Aguilera, 1990, p. 69).

Crisis related to perception that usual coping skills will be insufficient. "If in the appraisal process, the outcome is judged to be too overwhelming or too difficult to be dealt with using available coping skills, an individual is more likely to resort to the use of intrapsychic defensive mechanisms or distort the reality of the situation" (p. 69).

Crisis related to perceived lack of social support. "Confrontation with a stressful situation, combined with a lack of situational support, may lead to a state of disequilibrium and possible crisis" (p. 69).

Care Plan

A care plan based on Aguilera and Messick's theory of crisis intervention would focus on helping the client strengthen his or her problem-solving abilities. The problem solving process can be affected by a variety of internal and external factors. For example, the anxiety associated with problem solving increases as the value placed on finding a solution increases. This anxiety can serve both to stimulate and to impede problem solving, depending on it's severity. Some anxiety can help the client with intact problem-solving skills to mobilize resources by narrowing perceptions. Severe anxiety, on the other hand, can affect one's ability to concentrate on and thus comprehend the situation. In this context, the client is likely to be unable to make use of past experiences in finding solutions, and will need very structured guidance in identifying alternative solutions. Once identified, the client will need assistance in evaluating each alternative for potential success and in subsequently selecting which to implement. Examples of techniques utilized by the nurse might include, ". . .helping the individual to gain an intellectual understanding of the crisis or helping him to explore and ventilate his feelings. Other techniques may be helping the individual to find new and more effective coping mechanisms or utilizing other people as situational supports" (Aguilera, 1990, p. 64).

Perception of the Event

Aguilera (1990) contends that the emotional tension associated with a problem situation, as well as the coping behaviors employed to deal with it, are to an extent the result of one's perceptions (appraisal) of the situation. When an event is perceived as a threat to one's goals or values, emotional tension will follow. Based on the nature and degree of the threat, coping responses are initiated. Should the available coping resources be perceived as inadequate to resolve the threat, the emotional tension will continue to increase. The goal of reducing such emotional tension and associated symptoms is achieved through interventions aimed at helping the client establish a realistic perception (primary appraisal) of the event as well as his or her reservoir of available coping alternatives (secondary appraisal).

Situational Supports

The lack of available support persons to help solve the problem also contributes to the emotional tension associated with a problem situation. As social beings, individuals depend on meaningful relationships and interactions for their sense of value, self-worth, and confidence in the ability to achieve. Without adequate support in the context of a problem situation, individuals may be overwhelmed by a sense of vulnerability resulting in an increase in emotional tension. The goal of reducing such emotional tension can be reached through the implementation of interventions aimed at increasing the availability of persons that can help resolve the problem situation.

Available Coping Mechanisms

The effectiveness of one's available coping mechanisms can also contribute to the degree of emotional tension associated with a problem situation. In the context of a problem situation that has produced a degree of emotional tension, an individual will respond with behaviors that have been successful in reducing such tension in the past. Should such behaviors fail to reduce the tension, the degree of emotional tension felt by the individual will continue to increase. The goal of reducing this tension and its associated behaviors can be achieved through interventions aimed at identifying, teaching, and implementing new coping behaviors.

Implementation of the Care Plan

Implementation of the care plan involves techniques aimed at strengthening those balancing factors felt to be inadequate. The nurse facilitates the development of a realistic perception of the crisis event, available support systems, and/or new coping mechanisms.

Evaluation of the Care Plan

The effectiveness of the planned intervention is measured in terms of the degree of crisis resolution (product outcome evaluation). The reduction in psychological tension and return to usual level of functioning become hallmarks of crisis resolution. The nurse monitors the client's behavior for signs of reduced tension and psychological equilibrium. In addition, the nurse monitors the extent to which the nursing actions (process—nurse focused—evaluation) were carried out and the degree to which the etiology component is modified (process—client focused—evaluation).

THEORY-DIRECTED NURSING CARE FOR THE BROWN FAMILY

Aguilera and Messick's crisis intervention theory is applied to the Brown family. Each of the five steps of the nursing process are illustrated.

Assessing

The assessment data are organized under the categories of crisis, perception of the event, available situational support, and available coping mechanisms.

Crisis-Precipitating Event

Mary Brown and her unborn child are in critical condition in the MICU.

Crisis

The data relevant to the presence of psychological disequilibrium or crisis include the following: Mr. Brown is becoming dysfunctional, as evidenced by his excessive crying episodes, disturbances in eating and sleeping patterns, and lack of participation in decision making regarding his wife's care.

Perception of the Event

The data relevant to the perception of the event includes the following: Mr. Brown fears that they will both die (perceived threat); Mr. Brown believes that his wife's illness would have been minimized had he sought medical attention earlier and, thus, he is responsible for her possible death (distorted perception of the event).

Available Situational Support

The data relevant to the available situational support include the following: Mr. Brown's parents are very supportive and, since arranging for childcare for his son, have remained at the hospital; Mary's sisters, however, are not supportive and, in fact, have only negative interactions with him; furthermore, because of Mary's need for neuromuscular blockage, she is unable to interact with her husband (lack of situational support/negative support).

Available Coping Mechanisms

The data relevant to the available coping mechanisms include the following: Mr. Brown has never experienced the death of a close friend or family member before; Mr. Brown's usual method of dealing with major problems is that of withdrawal and avoidance; despite using these mechanisms, his emotional tension persists (inadequate available coping mechanisms).

Diagnosing

Although more than one nursing diagnose would be generated from the Brown data, only one is illustrated here. The following nursing diagnosis was formulated from the data presented in this case.

Crisis Related to Distorted Perception of the Event

The subjective and objective data that support the diagnosis are presented.

Response: Crisis

Subjective Data	**Objective Data**
"He just doesn't know what to do."	Mr. Brown has not slept in 3 days. Mr. Brown cries every time he visits his wife or thinks about her. Has not visited son. Does not talk to his wife. Does not initiate contact with staff.

Etiology: Distorted perception of the event

Subjective Data	**Objective Data**
"I'm sorry, Mary. Please don't die."	Parents report that he blames himself for not getting her to the doctor sooner.

Planning

The following goals and predicted outcomes have been formulated based on the response component of the nursing diagnosis, *crisis*.

Goal: Mr. Brown's crisis will be resolved.

Predicted Outcomes:

1. Mr. Brown will leave the hospital at night after the last visiting hour at least three times a week to sleep.
2. Mr. Brown will visit his son at least once a day.
3. Mr. Brown will talk to his wife during visiting hours.
4. Mr. Brown will make eye contact with the nursing staff and engage in conversation.
5. Mr. Brown will initiate appropriate conversation with medical and nursing staff regarding Mary's condition and response to treatment.
6. Mr. Brown's crying episodes will decrease.

Based on the etiology component of the nursing diagnosis statement, *distorted perception of the event*, the nursing interventions and nursing actions are planned.

Nursing Interventions:
Assist Mr. Brown in the development of a realistic perception regarding his actions and the severity of Mary's illness.

Nursing Actions	**Rationale**
1. Explain to Mr. Brown that viral infections often begin with non-specific symptoms which rapidly progress into more serious problems.	Helping the individual gain an understanding of the situation may elicit new coping (Aguilera, 1990).
2. Provide condition reports for Mr. Brown each time he visits Mary.	"As a result of the appraisal process coping behaviors are never static. They change constantly in both quality and degree as new information and cues are received during reappraisal activities" (Aguilera, 1990, p. 69).

3. Encourage Mr. Brown to ask questions about Mary's condition or treatment in order to understand the situation.

Planned interventions may involve "helping the individual to gain an intellectual understanding of the crisis or helping him to explore and ventilate his feelings" (Aguilera, 1990 p. 64).

Implementing

Ms. Johnson performed the planned nursing actions to facilitate the achievement of the client goal and predicted outcomes. She began by discussing with Mr. Brown the sequence of events that led to Mary's admission. During this discussion Ms. Johnson used her clarification skills to help Mr. Brown see that he could not have known of the seriousness of Mary's illness based on her initial complaints. She emphasized that the complaints associated with varicella, as well as other viral diseases, are often nonspecific and without obvious early warning signs. Praise was also provided for Mr. Brown's prompt action when Mary's condition deteriorated.

Ms. Johnson provided a brief explanation of all the equipment surrounding Mary's bed and discussed the treatment plan. During each visiting hour Ms. Johnson provided a progress report for Mr. Brown including any actual or expected changes in Mary's condition. Ms. Johnson stayed in the room during visiting hours long enough to give the progress report and answer any questions; she then provided privacy for Mr. Brown and his wife. Ms. Johnson encouraged Mr. Brown to touch his wife and talk to her while in the room so that she would know he was there. She also suggested that sometimes learning more about a situation can make it easier to deal with. She encouraged him to ask as many questions as he wanted to help him understand what was happening to Mary and what to expect.

Mr. Brown agreed that he had a lot of questions but felt overwhelmed by all of the machines in Mary's room and the "big words used by the doctors." Ms. Johnson reassured him that it was natural to be overwhelmed by all of the machines and the activity in an intensive care unit, but that the nursing staff and medical staff were eager to answer any questions.

Gradually Mr. Brown began asking questions during visiting hours. He eventually began using some of the medical terminology he was exposed to and knew all of the nurses by name. At one point he began asking questions about Mary's response to therapy described at previous visiting hours.

Evaluating

Product Evaluation

1. The first evening after Mr. Brown met with Ms. Johnson, he left the hospital and reported sleeping for about 7 hours. He slept the next night as well, but due to a change in Mary's condition he did not leave the hospital at night for the rest of the week. He did, however, take naps in the family room periodically between visiting hours.
2. Mr. Brown did visit his son every day, even on those days when he spent the night at the hospital.
3. On the first day Mr. Brown continued to sob at Mary's bedside, and he conversed very little. On the second day he began to cry less and talk more, telling her how much he loved her and missed her, and who had been there to visit.
4. By the second day Mr. Brown began addressing the nurses caring for Mary by name and made eye contact periodically.
5. By the end of the second day Mr. Brown would begin his visiting hour by asking if there had been any change in Mary's or the baby's condition. He would occasionally ask specific questions in regard to Mary's response to certain treatments.
6. Although on the third day Mary's condition deteriorated significantly, Mr. Brown appeared to be participating in the decision making with the physicians.

Process Evaluation

Nurse Focus (extent that planned nursing interventions and nursing actions were implemented).

- The nurse did assist Mr. Brown in his appraisal process through listening and clarification.
- The nurse provided short condition reports for Mr. Brown during each visiting hour. She also spoke with him on the phone on a few occasions when he called from home before the first visiting hour. The nurses on the night shift also provided condition reports during the night when he called.

Client Focus (extent that the etiology component of the nursing diagnosis statement was modified).

Mr. Brown did attempt to become an active participant in Mary's care by asking questions about her condition and treatment. He acknowledge the fact that he could not have known that Mary was critically ill based on her initial symptoms.

SUMMARY

This chapter has demonstrated the use of crisis intervention to assist a family to cope with the sudden critical illness of a family member. It illustrates that through strengthening the client's balancing factors, psychological equilibrium can be restored and thus, the crisis resolved.

REFERENCES

Aguilera, D. (1990). *Crisis intervention: Theory and methodology,* (6th ed.). St. Louis: C. V. Mosby.

Aguilera, D., & Messick, J. (1986). *Crisis Intervention: Theory and methodology,* (5th ed.). St. Louis: C. V. Mosby.

Caplan, G. (1964). *Principles of preventive psychiatry.* New York: Basic Books.

Hodovanic, B., Reardon, D., Reese, W., & Hedges, B. (1984). Family crisis intervention program in the medical intensive care unit. *Heart & Lung 13,* 243–249.

Lazarus, R., & Folkman, S. (1984). *Stress appraisal and coping.* New York: Springer Publishing Co.

Lindemann, E. (1944). Symptomatology and management of acute grief. *American Journal of Psychiatry, 101*(9), 141–148.

Chapter 3

Bandura's Social Cognitive Theory

Shirley Melat Ziegler, Wilda K. Arnold,
Susan Goad, Lois Hough,
Oneida Hughes, Rose Nieswiadomy,
and Gail Walden Watson

Nurses frequently assist clients and their families in changing patterns of behavior that are inadequate for sustaining or promoting health. The case of Harry Henderson and his wife will illustrate how the nurse can use Bandura's social cognitive theory to help clients learn and practice behaviors which will have a positive influence on their health.

Following the Henderson case presentation, three theories that might be used to guide theory-directed nursing care for the family are summarized. Then one of these theories, Bandura'a (1986) social cognitive theory, is selected for an in-depth demonstration of how Bandura's theory could be used to direct nursing care for the Henderson family.

CLIENT CASE

Harry Henderson is a 32-year-old white male trauma patient. His injuries, sustained in an auto accident, consist of a fracture of the right radius and ulna, multiple severed tendons of the left hand, and a lacerated trachea. The right arm is in a cast and the left hand is covered with a compression bandage. A Montgomery tube (a specialized form of T tube) is in place inside Mr. Henderson's trachea. The surgeon estimates that the Montgomery tube will be in place for 4 to 6 weeks.

During discharge planning Ms. Adams, the nurse, learned that the Henderson's live about 100 miles out of town in an area unserved by any type of home care agency. Further investigation revealed that Mrs. Henderson is the only possible care giver, once Mr. Henderson goes home.

Ms. Adams recalled the interactions she had observed between Mr. and Mrs. Henderson. They seemed to be an affectionate couple, holding hands frequently, welcoming the other's return after an absence, and smiling when making eye contact with each other. Mrs. Henderson readily performed feeding, mouth care, bathing, dressing, and toileting tasks for her husband. Mr. Henderson silently signaled gratitude for and satisfaction with the care he received from his wife. On the other hand Ms. Adams recalled that, whenever it was time for Mr. Henderson's tracheostomy care, Mrs. Henderson averted her eyes, began to fidget, and then abruptly left the room. Mr. Henderson's nurses had encouraged Mrs. Henderson to participate in the tracheostomy care. She consistently refused by saying, "I can't ever learn to do that." She also said "I don't want to have anything to do with that part of his care."

Ms. Adams approached Mrs. Henderson and discussed the need for her to learn to do tracheostomy care. "I just won't be able to do it," said Mrs. Henderson. She explained that when she was 16 years old, her mother had an extended period of illness and required considerable help with ordinary activities of daily living. Also, her mother had been totally dependent upon others for management of her colostomy.

As the only daughter, Mrs. Henderson was expected to give most of this care. She tried very hard to meet her mother's needs, apparently doing well enough with the maintenance tasks. However, whenever she worked with the colostomy, something always went wrong. Either she would soil her mother and the bed when removing a full bag or she would not put the clean bag on properly and it would leak. The experience of consistent mishaps associated with doing colostomy care had convinced Mrs. Henderson that she had no talent for giving any kind of complex nursing care. Mrs. Henderson went on to say, "When I have to take care of my husband's tracheostomy, it will be the same thing all over again."

PATTERNING CUES FROM CLIENT CASE

The nurse initiates the strategy for providing theory-directed nursing practice for the Henderson case, first by identifying the discrepancies in the case between the way the situation is and the way the situation should be. A discrepancy exists between Mr. Henderson's need for care upon discharge and Mrs. Henderson's ability to provide the needed care. Although Mrs. Henderson has learned to provide most of the care her husband will need, she has refused to learn to care for his tracheostomy. Using the reasoning process of induction, Ms. Adams identifies the following cues:

- The Hendersons are an affectionate couple.
- Mrs. Henderson provides most of her husband's care needs.
- Mr. Henderson shows gratitude to his wife.
- Mrs. Henderson does not observe the tracheostomy procedure and refuses to participate in the procedure.

Organizing these cues into a pattern, Ms. Adams realizes she is faced with the problem of how to help Mrs. Henderson change her behavior pattern of refusing to provide tracheostomy care for her husband to the behavior pattern of skillfully providing tracheostomy care. The nurse is confronted with both teaching Mrs. Henderson how to provide her husband's care and determining why she has been reluctant to both learn and perform the tracheostomy care. The next step in the strategy for theory-directed nursing is the linking of the identified pattern from the case data to the theories stored in long-term memory.

SELECTED RELEVANT THEORIES

A number of theories could be used in providing care for Mr. Henderson and his family. Three theories will be considered in order to illustrate that different theories provide different explanations for Mrs. Henderson's behavior, leading to different etiologies for the nursing diagnoses and, therefore, different nursing interventions. The theories considered are rational-emotive therapy theory (Ellis, 1973), behavioral theory (Wolpe, 1973), and social cognitive theory (Bandura, 1971, 1977a, 1977b, 1978, 1982, 1986).

Rational-Emotive Therapy Theory

One theory that might be considered for this case situation is the rational-emotive therapy theory (RET) of Ellis (1973). RET is based on the premise that individuals control their own lives by the way they interpret events that occur in their lives and by the actions they choose to take based on their beliefs. Ellis used the acronym ABC to indicate the main concepts of his theory. A is the *a*ctivating event, B is the person's *b*elief about A, and C represents the emotional *c*onsequences of the belief system.

RET hypothesizes the conclusion that A directly causes C. In actuality it is B, an irrational belief about A, that causes the distress at point C. In the case of Mrs. Henderson, when she attempted to provide colostomy care for her mother (A), she felt like a failure (C). Therefore, her belief (B) is that she will not be able to provide adequate tracheostomy care for her husband.

The nursing diagnosis generated from this theory is "refusal to perform tracheostomy care related to the irrational belief that she is incapable of performing the procedure." First, nursing interventions for Mrs. Henderson would be focused on changing her irrational beliefs concerning her inability to provide tracheostomy care for her husband. Then, she would need to be taught the technical aspects of tracheostomy care.

The difficulty the nurse would encounter in using RET in this case is that the theory does not address the acquisition of psychomotor skills. Therefore, this theory may not be the most desirable theory for the nurse to use in working with Mrs. Henderson.

Wolpe's Behavioral Theory

Another theory that might be considered for this case situation would be Wolpe's (1973) behavioral theory. According to this theory, anxiety is the generator of behavior, with a hierarchical relationship (anxiety hierarchy) being established among anxiety-producing stimuli. Thus, the focus of this theory is on reducing anxiety, thereby enabling more acceptable behaviors to be substituted for maladaptive behavior.

One of the treatment techniques used by behaviorists in helping individuals cope with anxiety is that of systematic desensitization. The individual is taught to relax and then, over many sessions, is presented with progressively more threatening situations. Thus, anxiety is extinguished in a hierarchical fashion, from the lowest to the highest level of anxiety.

Mrs. Henderson's experience in caring for her mother's colostomy was the anxiety-producing stimulus. The anxiety produced by this experience has caused Mrs. Henderson to avoid taking care of her husband's tracheostomy. The anxiety generated by this experience is seemingly high in the anxiety hierarchy. Thus, the nursing diagnosis generated from this theory is "refusal to perform tracheostomy care related to dysfunctional anxiety".

The nursing intervention for Mrs. Henderson would be that of systematic desensitization. First, she would be taught relaxation techniques. After she had learned to relax, she would be introduced to the care of the tracheostomy in a progressive, step-by-step fashion.

Although this intervention would change Mrs. Henderson's behavior, it would likely take several weeks because the lower levels of anxiety would need to be alleviated before the higher levels could be addressed. In addition to the time constriction, each member of the nursing staff would have to be knowledgeable and capable of implementing the desensitization technique on a 24-hour basis.

Bandura's Social Cognitive Theory

Bandura's (1986) social cognitive theory provides a framework for analyzing human motivation, thought, and action from a social cognitive perspective. Social cognitive theory embraces an interactional model in which environmental events, personal factors, and behavior all operate as interacting determinants of each other. Social cognitive theory considers both how behavioral patterns are acquired (learned) and how patterns of behaviors, once learned, are regulated (how the behavior either continues to be performed or is discontinued). In social cognitive theory, psychological functioning is seen as a continuous reciprocal interaction between behavior and its controlling conditions. Behavior is learned by directly experiencing response consequences or through observation of other peoples' behaviors and its consequences for them. Emotional responses are also observationally learned. Behavior is both insightful and foresightful. The cognitive capacity of individuals allows them to solve problems symbolically without having to enact the various alternatives and to foresee the probable consequences of different actions. Thus, people are capable of regulating their own behavior. Because Bandura's theory provides an explanation for why Mrs. Henderson is reluctant to learn the behavior in the first place, and provides guidelines regarding how to teach her the needed psychomotor tasks, it has been selected for illustration in this client situation.

DESCRIPTION OF BANDURA'S SOCIAL COGNITIVE THEORY

Bandura's (1986) social cognitive theory is frequently referred to as social learning theory. However, Bandura renamed it social cognitive theory in his 1986 publication in the belief that the scope of the theory was broader than the original label had described. The theory is concerned with such psychosocial phenomena as motivation and self-regulatory mechanisms that extend beyond the concept of learning. Also, Bandura stated that the name "social cognitive theory" would help the reader to distinguish this theory from several others that are called social learning theories, such as Rotter's 1954 theory, Dollard and Miller's 1950 theory, and Patterson's 1982 theory (as cited in Bandura, 1986).

The reader is reminded that the description of Bandura's theory is brief because of space limitations. It is assumed that those who wish to utilize Bandura's theory will seek out additional sources (especially primary sources) that describe the theory in detail. Major primary sources (listed in the reference section) include publications by Bandura in 1971, 1977a, 1977b, 1978, 1982, and 1986. Secondary sources, in which Bandura's theory is presented in the context of nursing, include Erikson, Tomlin, and Swain (1983), Hall and Smith (1985), and Lowe (1991). Bandura's theory is complex and addresses multiple concepts. The authors, therefore, have selected those concepts they believe are the most pertinent to the case presentation. These selected concepts are named and theoretically defined, with clinical examples identified and major relational statements presented.

Major Concepts

The selected concepts of Bandura's theory can be organized under the two major phenomena that this theory addresses: the acquisition of behavior and the regulation (or continued performance) of behavior. The major concept of Bandura's social cognitive theory concerned with the acquisition of behavior is modeling. The major concept of Bandura's social cognitive theory concerned with the regulation of behavior is reinforcement. Table 3.1 presents a summary of these two major concepts and their selected subconcepts. The selected subconcepts are classified under the acquisition of behavior (modeling) and the regulation of behavior (reinforcement).

Table 3.1 Selected concepts of Bandura's Social Cognitive Theory classified under the acquisition of behavior (modeling) and the regulation of behavior (reinforcement)

ACQUISITION OF BEHAVIOR—Modeling
  Attentional Processes
    Model Charateristics
    Observer Characteristics
  Retention Processes
    Imaginal
    Verbal
    Symbolic (cognitive) rehearsal
    Motor rehearsal
  Motor Reproduction Processes
REGULATION OF BEHAVIOR—Reinforcement
  External (Direct) Reinforcement
  Vicarious Reinforcement
  Self (Internal) Reinforcement
    Outcome expectancy
    Efficacy expectation
      Performance accomplishments
      Vicarious experience
      Verbal persuasion
      Emotional arousal

Theoretical Definitions of Major Concepts

Modeling

Modeling refers to a process of transmitting information to the observer that elicits the observer's responses. Three interrelated concepts are involved in modeling: attentional processes, retention processes, and motor reproduction.

1. *Attentional processes* refer to the observer's attention to and recognition of the essential features of a model's behavior. The attentional process consists of two concepts: modeling stimuli and observer characteristics.
   a. *modeling stimuli* refers to the characteristics of the model, such as interpersonal attractiveness.
   b. *observer characteristics* refers to the observer's attributes, such as sensory and motor capacities.

2. *Retention processes* refer to the observer's retention of the activities that have been modeled into long-term memory. There are four concepts (systems) associated with retention: imaginal, verbal, symbolic rehearsal, and motor rehearsal.

   a. The *imaginal* system concerns the use of mental images of the observed behavior.

   b. The *verbal* system concerns the use of words or symbols to code the information into memory.

   c. The *symbolic (cognitive) rehearsal* system concerns the observer's mental rehearsal of a modeled behavior.

   d. The *motor rehearsal* system concerns the observer's motor rehearsal of a modeled behavior.

3. *Motor reproduction processes* refer to the observer's reproduction of the modeled behavior.

Reinforcement

People do not enact everything they learn. They may acquire all of the capabilities to carry out behavior but rarely or never perform them. Once behavior is learned, the regulation of behavior relies on the motivational process (incentive) of reinforcement. Behavior is extensively controlled by its consequences.

Reinforcement refers to the consequences of behavior and can influence behavior by creating expectations of similar outcomes in the future. There are three concepts which address the source of reinforcement: external reinforcement, vicarious reinforcement, and self-reinforcement.

1. *external reinforcement (or direct reinforcement)* refers to the process in which behavior is controlled by its immediate consequences.

2. *vicarious reinforcement* refers to a process in which one witnesses the rewards and punishments of others and thus alters one's actions based on these observations.

3. *self-reinforcement or internal reinforcement* refers to a self-produced, self-monitored process in which individuals enhance and maintain their own behavior by rewarding themselves with rewards they control whenever they attain self-prescribed standards. Two concepts are involved in self-reinforcement: outcome expectancy and efficacy expectation.

   a. *Outcome expectancy* refers to a person's estimate that a given behavior is capable of bringing about a desired outcome.

   b. *Efficacy expectation* refers to a person's conviction that a behavior can be performed in a manner that will produce a desired outcome. There are four concepts which address the source of efficacy expectation: performance accomplishment, vicarious experience, verbal persuasion, and emotional arousal.

- *Performance accomplishment* refers to personal experiences that result in successful outcomes.

- *Vicarious experience* refers to the observation of a model performing threatening activities without adverse consequences.

- *Verbal persuasion* refers to expectations created through another person's verbal message. The message encourages the individual to believe that a behavior can be performed successfully, even if the task appears to be overwhelming.

- *Emotional arousal* refers to a cognitive process aimed at reducing avoidance behavior by leading individuals "to believe that the things they have previously feared no longer affect them internally" (Bandura, 1977a, p. 82).

Examples of Concepts Relevant to Clinical Practice

Clinical examples for the concepts classified under modeling (acquisition of behavior) and reinforcement (regulation of behavior) are presented.

Modeling (Acquisition of Behavior)

The teacher of CPR first gets the attention (attentional process) of the students by presenting a short video depicting an adolescent falling to the ground after touching a high voltage wire. The adolescent is not breathing; there is no pulse. The teacher talks about the significance of maintaining circulatory and respiratory functions, while simultaneously demonstrating CPR for students. The students store mental images (retention process-imaginal) of how the procedure is physically performed. The students also store in memory the steps of the procedures in the correct order (retention process-verbal). The students then practice, in their minds, the steps of the procedure and imagine themselves performing CPR. Finally the students practice the steps of CPR (retention process-motor rehearsal). After sufficient rehearsal, the students demonstrate CPR to the teacher (motor reproduction).

Reinforcement (Regulation of Behavior)

While the students wait for an opportunity to return the demonstration, the students observe the teacher praising some students for an excellent performance and pointing out to other students the areas in which the performance needs to be improved (vicarious reinforcement). The students practice CPR until they believe they will be able to perform CPR adequately in the evaluation demonstration (self-reinforcement). During the performance evaluation the teacher congratulates each student for an accurate CPR performance saying, "You have successfully performed CPR" (external reinforcement). The teacher then shows the ending of the videotape, which depicts a healthy adolescent several weeks after the electrical shock. The observation of the successful results of CPR is an additional example of vicarious reinforcement.

Major Relational Statements

The relational statements that serve to link the major concepts are presented. *Modeling* (the acquisition of behavior) and *reinforcement* (the regulation of behavior) again serve as the major concepts.

Bandura points out that behavior is learned (acquired) before it is performed. Learning takes place from a teacher (a model) who repeatedly:

1) demonstrates (models) the desired responses (attentional processes and retention processes)
2) instructs the learner to reproduce the desired responses (retention processes and motor reproduction processes)
3) prompts the behavior when it fails to occur (attention, retention, and motor reproduction processes).

Bandura believes that this approach to teaching will eventually elicit the desired responses in most people.

Relational statements, concerned with the regulation of behavior, follow. People are not only affected by the experiences created by their own actions (external reinforcement), they also regulate their behavior on the basis of observed consequences (vicarious reinforcement), as well as those they create for themselves (self-reinforcement). People fear and tend to avoid threatening situations they believe exceed their coping skills; they get involved when they judge themselves capable of handling situations. Efficacy expectations are a major determinant of people's choice of activities, how much effort they will expend, and how long they will sustain an effort in dealing with stressful situations. Of the four major sources of information used for efficacy expectations, performance-accomplishment based sources of information are superior in changing behavior when compared to vicarious experience, verbal persuasion, and emotional arousal.

IMPLICATIONS OF BANDURA'S SOCIAL COGNITIVE THEORY FOR CLINICAL PRACTICE

This section presents the use of Bandura's theory in nursing practice. Factors to be assessed, methods of assessing, theory-specific diagnoses, care planning, and evaluation of care are presented.

Factors to be Assessed and Methods of Assessing

The major concepts of Bandura's theory make up the factors to be assessed. First, the degree to which the desired behavior has been acquired and the conditions under which the behavior was acquired are assessed. Assessment will include the attentional processes (relevant characteristics of both the model and the observer), the retention processes of the observer (imaginal, verbal, symbolic rehearsal, and motor rehearsal), and the observer's ability to reproduce the modeled behavior. Next, reinforcement factors will be assessed regarding the level of external, vicarious, and self-reinforcement (internal) standards. The outcome expectancy of the client regarding the desired behavior will be assessed as well as the client's efficacy expectation. Finally, the sources of the client's efficacy expectations (performance accomplishments, vicarious experience, verbal persuasion, and emotional arousal) are assessed.

Social cognitive theory is based on the premise that both people and their environment are reciprocal determinants of each other. Therefore, theory-based assessment will include methods of assessing the client and the environment. Methods of obtaining data include direct interviewing of the individual and observation of the interactions of the individual with reference groups and others in the environment whose judgement he/she values. No specific assessment tool has been generated to assess a client using Bandura's social cognitive theory. Such an assessment tool needs to be generated and its psychometric qualities determined.

Theory-Specific Diagnoses

Sample nursing diagnoses are presented that are specific to Bandura's social cognitive theory. They focus on the primary determinants of observational learning.

Response Component

Bandura's theory is helpful in generating a number of response components for use in generating theory-specific nursing diagnoses. Examples of behaviors that may be included in the response component of the nursing diagnosis statement are: anxiety, behaviors inappropriate to role expectations, low self-esteem, depression, chronic discouragement, feelings of worthlessness, lack of purposefulness, excessive self-disparagement, failures in learning, performance failures (knows how to perform but does not perform), deviant behaviors (against social norms), and refusal to perform health promoting behaviors.

Etiology Component

Etiology components for the nursing diagnoses statements could reflect problems arising in the acquisition of behavior or in the regulation of behavior. Examples of etiologies that may arise during the acquisition of behavior include:

1. The behavior is inadequately modeled.
2. The learner may fail to observe the relevant activities for performing the desired behavior.
3. The learner inadequately codes the modeled events for memory representation.
4. The model has low prestige to the learner.
5. The learner does not value the consequences of the behavior (the reinforcement).
6. The learner lacks the requisite psychomotor skills.
7. The learner receives inadequate feedback regarding performance.

Examples of etiologies that may arise in the regulation of behavior include:

1. The standards for self-evaluation (self-reinforcement system) may be unrealistically high or low.
2. The environment does not value the learned behavior and thus the behavior is not initiated.
3. The learner may fail to learn rewarding methods of controlling the environment, that is, behavior with functional value in influencing a favorable response in others.
4. The learner has inadequate incentives for performing the behaviors.
5. The learner may inappropriately associate an unrelated event to a traumatic event (conditioned aversive stimuli).

Sample Nursing Diagnoses

A selection from the response and etiology examples, generated from Bandura's theory, was used to generate the following examples of nursing diagnoses.

1. *Anxiety related to inappropriate association of loss of personal control with the fear of flying.*
   "Events that happen to occur in the context of a traumatic experience but are in no way causally related to them sometimes take on aversive properties and produce inappropriate generalizations of anxiety reactions" (Bandura, 1971, p. 16).

2. *Feelings of worthlessness related to stringent standards selected as indices for positive self-reinforcement.*

   "Self-esteem is the result of discrepancies between a person's behavior and the standards that he has selected as indices of personal merit" (Bandura, 1971, p. 31).

3. *Inability to solicit help from others related to inadequate knowledge of how to bring about desired response from others.*

   Problem-prone individuals may possess aversive styles of behavior that predictably produce negative social climates wherever they go; people play an active role in constructing their own reinforcement contingencies through their characteristic mode of response (Bandura, 1971, p. 40).

4. *Stealing related to antisocial conditions of reinforcement.*

   "Most of the behaviors that people display are learned, either deliberately, or inadvertently, through the influence of example" (Bandura, 1971, p. 5). If a child observes stealing as a rewarded behavior in the environment, the stealing behavior is likely to be modeled.

5. *Failure to learn health-promoting behaviors related to deficits in long-term memory.*

   "If one is to reproduce a model's behavior when the latter is no longer present to serve as a guide, the response patterns must be represented in memory. . ." (Bandura, 1971, p. 7).

6. *Inappropriate standards of achievement set for self related to the adherence to standards of achievement possessed before loss in ability following physical injury.*

   ". . . an individual may be unable to coordinate various actions in the required pattern and sequence because of physical limitations" (Bandura, 1971, p. 8).

Care Plan

A care plan based on Bandura's social cognitive theory would focus on helping the client learn new behavior through modeling or learning to modify dysfunctional behavior through changing the anticipated reinforcement. Thus, the learning of behaviors or modification of behaviors occurs in a social learning context through two factors: 1) social models and 2) differential reinforcement.

Learning New Behaviors (Acquisition of Behavior)

Bandura (1977a) differentiates between the acquisition of behavior and the performance of behavior because people do not display every idea they learn. Behavior is acquired primarily through observational learning. Behavior is taught primarily through a process Bandura termed modeling.

The functions of modeling are to teach component skills and provide the rules for organizing them into new structures of behavior or to reorganize components skills already learned. Models can serve as instructors, inhibitors, disinhibitors, facilitators, stimulus enhancers, and emotion arousers (Bandura, 1986, p. 51). The relative effectiveness of the different methods of modeling depends on the developmental competence of observers and the complexity and codability of the modeled activities.

For example, in cognitive modeling, the models provide the rules and strategies that guide their choice of behavior; this approach is essentially a deductive one. On the other hand, in behavioral modeling, the models provide examples for inducing rules and strategies; this approach is primarily an inductive one. Both cognitive and behavioral modeling are usually needed as guides. People can acquire abstract principles from cognitive modeling but remain uncertain about how to implement them if they have not had examples (behavioral modeling). Thus, behavioral modeling combined with rule verbalization is usually more effective than either alone in promoting rule-governed behavior (Bandura, 1986, p. 101). For example, a person could be told the steps to follow in performing an injection in a muscle. However, a demonstration is needed to show the actual performance of the skill.

Bandura distinguishes between knowledge and skill. Knowing a rule and how to perform a desired behavior does not ensure optimal performance. Performance skills require transforming knowledge into skilled action. Observational learning cannot be reflected at the behavioral level until the necessary physical maturation has occurred. Thus, an important component in the acquisition of knowledge is practice of the behavior.

Just as the characteristics or capabilities of the learner are important, so are the characteristics of the teacher. The nurse needs to be cognizant of how she or he is perceived by the client. "When people are uncertain about the wisdom of modeled courses of actions, they must rely on such cues as general appearance, speech, style, age, symbols of socioeconomic success, and signs of expertise as indicators of probable success" (Bandura, 1986, p. 208). Bandura (1977a) observed that perceptive and confident people emulate both idealized models and those whose behavior is highly useful. The attributes of models exert the greatest influence when it is unclear what consequences the observer's behavior is likely to have. Therefore, the probable value of modeled behavior must be judged from appearances and signs of achievement of the model.

Modification of Behavior (Regulation of Behavior)

Self-referent thought mediates the relationship between knowledge and action (Bandura, 1986, p. 390). Interventions to modify dysfunctional behavior primarily involve the alteration of the client's beliefs regarding the level and strength of self-efficacy (Bandura, 1977b). Changes in the client's behavior result from diverse modes of intervention. Interventions serve as a means of strengthening the expectations of personal efficacy. Any given intervention may draw on one or more of the four sources of information utilized to form expectations of personal efficacy (performance accomplishments, vicarious experience, verbal persuasion, and emotional arousal). Modes of intervention for each of the four sources of information are presented.

If the intervention is designed to focus on the first source of information, performance accomplishments, the nurse assists the client in repeated successes in order to reduce the negative impact of occasional failures. Other modes of induction include participant modeling, performance desensitization, performance exposure, and self-instructed performance. For example, performance desensitization could be used with phobics to visualize themselves in progressively threatening activities. The nurse intervenes using participant modeling by structuring the environment so clients can perform successfully despite their incapacities. Examples that can be used by the nurse include graduated tasks and joint performances of the task (such as tracheostomy care) with the nurse.

Clients also rely on vicarious experience as a source of efficacy information. Interventions include live and symbolic modeling. When clients observe the nurse perform activities perceived as threatening without harmful consequences, they will receive encouragement that they too can perform activities without fear of harmful consequences. Vicarious experience is less dependable, however, than direct evidence of personal accomplishments.

The nurse can also employ verbal persuasion. The client can be led by suggestion into coping successfully with a new task or problem situation. This method of intervention is also weaker than those arising from self-accomplishment because it is not authentic experientially for the client.

Social persuasion techniques are a more effective intervention if the provisional aids for effective actions are also provided by the nurse.

Emotional arousal is another source of information that can affect perceived self-efficacy. Modes of induction include attribution, relaxation, symbolic desensitization, and symbolic exposure. Nurses can intervene by use of progressive muscle relaxation techniques to help decrease the disruptive emotion associated with a behavior.

Implementation of the Care Plan

Implementation of the care plan is a balancing of the increments of the behavior to be learned with the associated efficacy expectations. The nurse manages learning conditions so that success is experienced more often than failure during performance of the incremental sequence. Sequential successes foster the expectation that mastery of the total performance will be achieved.

Evaluation of the Care Plan

Mastery based on weak expectations is quickly extinguished. Mastery based on strong expectations perseveres. This relationship between strength of expectation and persistence of performance forms the basis for evaluation. The nurse monitors the client's ongoing behavior to determine whether or not the desired performance persists.

THEORY-DIRECTED NURSING CARE FOR THE HENDERSON CASE

Bandura's social cognitive theory is applied to the Henderson family. Each of the five steps of the nursing process are illustrated.

Assessing

The assessment data are organized under the categories of acquisition of behavior and regulation of behavior. The following assessment data is relevant to the acquisition of behavior. Mrs. Henderson is the only care giver available once Mr. Henderson goes home. She has readily provided the activities of daily living care for Mr. Henderson. However, Mrs. Henderson has not learned to provide her husband's tracheostomy care. In fact, she abruptly leaves the room when the care is provided (dysfunctional attentional process). Until the nurse can secure Mrs. Henderson's attention, she cannot model the desired behavior, nor can Mrs. Henderson learn tracheostomy care. There are no data suggesting that Mrs. Henderson lacks the ability to memorize the steps of tracheostomy care or that she lacks the motor skills to carry out the procedure.

The following assessment data is relevant to the regulation of behavior. The data reveal that Mrs. Henderson is experiencing difficulty in the regulatory aspects of her behavior. The history of her failures while giving colostomy care to her mother (negative external reinforcement), her comments regarding her expectation that she will not be able to do it (self-reinforcement, specifically her level of efficacy expectation), and her refusal to stay in the room and observe the care (lack of opportunity for observing vicarious reinforcement) provide the assessment data regarding her difficulty in the regulation of her behavior. There are no data suggesting that she believes the tracheostomy care is unnecessary (outcome expectation). Mrs. Henderson has indicated that she believes that tracheostomy care will promote her husband's well-being. She appears to fear, and thus avoid, the tracheostomy care situation because she believes the requirements exceed her abilities. Her husband has provided her with positive external reinforcement regarding the activities of daily living that she has readily provided for him.

Diagnosing

The following diagnosis was formulated based on the data presented in the clinical case.

Avoidance of Performing Tracheostomy Care Related to Expectation that the Care will be Performed Inadequately

The subjective and objective data that support the diagnosis are presented.

Response: Avoidance of performing tracheostomy care

Subjective Data	**Objective Data**
"I don't want to have anything to do with that part of his care."	Refuses to provide tracheostomy part of his care. Averts eyes and leaves room when tracheostomy care is done.

Etiology: Expectation that care will be performed inadequately

Subjective Data	**Objective Data**
"When I have to take care of my husband's tracheostomy, it will be the same thing all over again." "I just won't be able to do it".	Report of poor experience with giving colostomy care.

Planning

Based on the response component of the nursing diagnosis, *avoidance of performing tracheostomy care,* goals and predicted outcomes have been formulated.

Goal: Mrs. Henderson will perform tracheostomy care successfully
Predicted Outcomes:

1. Mrs. H. will observe the nurse performing tracheostomy care for one day.
2. After 2 days Mrs. H. will perform tracheostomy care with the nurse's assistance.
3. After 4 days Mrs. H. will independently perform the tracheostomy care while the nurse watches.
4. Upon discharge from the hospital Mrs. H. will independently perform the tracheostomy care for her husband.

Based on the etiology component of the nursing diagnosis statement, *expectation that care will be provided inadequately,* the nursing interventions and nursing actions are planned.

Nursing Interventions:
Strengthen Mrs. Henderson's beliefs regarding her personal efficacy to produce the outcome expectation of a healthful outcome for her husband. The nurse will assist Mrs. Henderson to change her expectation of her own performance by teaching her the technique of tracheostomy care and reinforcing her performance.

Nursing Actions	**RATIONALE**
1. Praise Mrs. H. for the care she has provided for her husband.	"In attempts to influence behavior verbal persuasion is widely used because of its ease and ready availability" (Bandura, 1977a, p. 82).
2. Discuss with Mrs. H. her experience with her mother's colostomy and the opportunities she was offered at that time to learn this skill.	"People are led, through persuasive suggestion, into believing they can cope successfully with what has overwhelmed them in the past" (Bandura, 1977a, p. 82.).
3. Plan with Mrs. H. the timing of and the type of learning opportunities she will need to learn tracheostomy care.	"By managing the stimulus determinants of given activities and producing consequences for their own actions, people are able to control their own behavior to some degree" (Bandura, 1977a, p. 3).
4. Provide an opportunity for Mrs. H. to talk with other individuals who have provided tracheostomy care for relatives by introducing them to her.	"The impact of verbal persuasion on self-efficacy will vary depending on the perceived credibility of persuaders" (Bandura, 1977a, p. 202.).
5. Provide a video on tracheostomy care for Mrs. H. to view and discuss.	"Information can be conveyed by physical pictorial representation, or verbal description" (Bandura, 1977a, p. 39).
6. Nurse will perform tracheostomy care on Mr. H. with the wife observing.	"Man's capacity to learn by observation enables him to acquire large units of behavior by example without having to build up the patterns gradually by tedious trial and error" (Bandura, 1977a, p. 2).

7. Mrs. H. will assist the nurse in performing tracheostomy care for her husband.

"Through participant modeling it is possible to achieve rapid reality testing, which provides the corrective experience for change" (Bandura, 1977a, p. 83).

8. Mrs. H. provides tracheostomy care for Mr. H., while the nurse observes her performance and gives feedback on those steps which Mrs. H. performs successfully.

"Performance accomplishments provide the most dependable source of efficacy expectations because they are based on one's personal experience" Bandura, 1977a, p. 81).

9. The nurse redemonstrates the steps of tracheostomy care that were difficult for Mrs. H. to perform.

"A model who repeatedly demonstrates desired response, instructs others to reproduce the behavior, prompts them physically when they succeed, may eventually produce matching responses in most people" (Bandura, 1977a, p. 29).

10. Elicit from Mrs. H. her expectancy of future successes.

"The greater the increments in self-perceived efficacy, the greater the changes in behavior" (Bandura, 1971, p. 206).

Implementing

The nurse performed the planned nursing actions to facilitate the achievement of the client goal and predicted outcomes. Initially the nurse praised Mrs. Henderson for the skills that she demonstrated as she provided the activities of daily living for Mr. Henderson. In addition, it was pointed out that Mr. Henderson indicated his satisfaction with the readiness and efficacy with which his wife provided this care. The nurse empathized with Mrs. Henderson regarding the past experiences in providing colostomy care for her mother and emphasized that people may fail in attempting to provide skilled nursing procedures because they have been given an inadequate opportunity to learn the skill.

Mrs. Henderson and the nurse discussed the proposed teaching plan for preparing her to give tracheostomy care for Mr. Henderson. She was offered the opportunity to talk with other people who performed the same care for their relatives, but Mrs. Henderson declined and this step in the plan was eliminated. The next phase of the plan consisted of allowing Mrs. Henderson to become familiar and comfortable with the equipment necessary for the care and the procedure itself. This was accomplished in a simulated setting provided by the nurse who praised Mrs. Henderson's efforts and waited for her to signify that she was ready for the next step of the teaching plan.

After the simulated preparation, Mrs. Henderson watched a videotape illustrating how the tracheostomy care was to be performed, with the nurse available to answer any questions or address any of Mrs. Henderson's concerns. After discussing the procedure with the nurse, Mrs. Henderson wanted to review the videotape again.

At this time Mrs. Henderson indicated a readiness to continue and observed the nurse perform the tracheostomy care on Mr. Henderson. Mrs. Henderson asked a number of questions and, later, again observed the nurse providing the care.

The next day the nurse suggested that Mrs. Henderson assist in providing the tracheostomy care. Mrs. Henderson was hesitant to do so and asked to observe one more time, which she did. The next time the procedure was performed, Mrs. Henderson assisted and the nurse praised her for what she accomplished.

Mrs. Henderson then agreed that she was ready to attempt the tracheostomy care with the nurse present. The care was provided, with the nurse assisting when necessary. Upon completion of the task, the nurse and Mrs. Henderson discussed what had occurred and again the nurse praised Mrs. Henderson. They also planned for Mrs. Henderson to complete the procedure with the nurse present but offering no assistance. Continuing in this fashion, by the fifth day of instruction, Mrs. Henderson was able to perform the care without nursing assistance.

Evaluating

Product Evaluation (Extent that Goals and Predicted Outcomes were Met)

1. On the first day Mrs. Henderson became familiar with the equipment and observed the nurse perform the task in a simulated setting. In addition, she viewed the videotape two times.
2. On the second day Mrs. Henderson observed the nurse providing thetracheostomy care two times. Mrs. Henderson was hesitant to

assist the nurse with the procedure and asked to wait until the next day. She again observed the nurse perform the task.

3. On the third day she decided that she would be able to assist the nurse with the procedure and did so several times.
4. On the fourth day Mrs. Henderson provided the care, with the nurse assisting two times. Then Mrs. Henderson provided the care with the nurse present, but not assisting with the procedure.
5. By the fifth day Mrs. Henderson was able to provide the tracheostomy care without nursing assistance.
6. After discharge, a follow-up phone call revealed that Mrs. Henderson had been providing the tracheostomy care without incident.

Process Evaluation

Nurse Focus (extent that planned nursing interventions and nursing actions were implemented).
1. The nurse did not provide the opportunity for Mrs. Henderson to talk with other individuals who had provided tracheostomy care for relatives because Mrs. Henderson requested that this not be done.
2. The nurse did demonstrate tracheostomy care in the simulated lab and provided a videotape for Mrs. Henderson to watch.
3. The nurse demonstrated tracheostomy care on Mr. Henderson, with Mrs. Henderson observing.
4. The nurse observed Mrs. Henderson providing tracheostomy care and praised her for her efforts.

Client Focus (extent that etiology component of the nursing diagnosis statement was modified).
1. The client verbalized that she felt competent to provide her husband's tracheostomy care when he was discharged.
2. She offered to talk with other caregivers regarding her initial reluctance to provide the care and her subsequent success is learning the care.

SUMMARY

This section described and applied social cognitive theory, in the context of the nursing process, to a family case. The application of Bandura's social cognitive theory to the family case demonstrates that "by arranging environmental inducements, generating cognitive supports and producing consequences for their own actions, people are able to exercise some measure of control over their own behavior" (Bandura, 1977a, p. 12).

REFERENCES

Bandura, A. (1971). *Social learning theory*. Morristown, NJ: General Learning Press.

Bandura, A. (1977a). *Social learning theory*. Englewood Cliff, NJ: Prentice-Hall.

Bandura, A. (1977b). Self-efficacy: Toward a unifying theory of behavioral change. *Psychological Review, 84*(2), 191–215.

Bandura, A. (1978). The self system in reciprocal determinism. *American Psychologist, 33*, 344–358.

Bandura, A. (1982). Self-efficacy mechanism in human agency. *American Psychologist, 37*, 122–147.

Bandura, A. (1986). *Social foundations of thought and action: A social cognitive theory*. Englewood Cliffs, NJ: Prentice-Hall.

Ellis, A. (1973). *Humanistic psychotherapy: The rational emotive approach*. New York: McGraw-Hill

Erickson, H. C., Tomlin, E., & Swain, M. A. (1983). *Modeling and role modeling: A theory and paradigm for nursing*. Englewood Cliffs, NJ: Prentice-Hall.

Hall, L., & Smith, N. (1985). *Self care nursing: Promotion of health*. Englewood Cliffs, NJ: Prentice-Hall.

Lowe, N. K. (1991). Maternal confidence in coping with labor: A self-effiacy concept. *Journal of Gynecological Nursing, 20*, 457–463.

Wolpe, J. (1973). *The practice of behavior therapy* (2nd ed.). New York: Pergamon Press.

SUGGESTED READINGS

Ellis, A. (1987). *The practice of rational-emotive therapy (RET)*. New York: Springer Publishing Co.

Ellis, A., & Grieger, R. (Eds.) (1977). *Handbook of rational-emotive therapy*. New York: Springer Publishing Co.

Wolpe, J. (1986). Individualization: The categorical imperative behavior therapy practice. *Journal of Behavior Therapy and Experimental Psychiatry, 17*(3), 145–153.

Chapter 4

Beck's Cognitive Theory of Depression

Shirley Melat Ziegler

At least 12% of the U.S. adult population have had, or will have, an episode of depression requiring treatment (Beck, Rush, Shaw, & Emery, 1979). In fact, depression is a common response to problems experienced with health, such as chronic illness. It is estimated that 20 to 60% of ambulatory medical patients are depressed (Dreyfus, 1988). The case of Mrs. Moon will illustrate how the nurse can use theory to help clients deal with depression as a response to a health problem.

Following the Moon case presentation, three theories that might be selected to guide theory-directed nursing care for Mrs. Moon are summarized. Then one of these theories, Beck's (Beck et al., 1979) cognitive theory of depression, is selected for an in-depth demonstration of how a theory could be used to direct nursing care for Mrs. Moon.

CLIENT CASE

Mrs. Moon is a 42-year-old white married middle-class woman who was recently treated surgically for an intrauterine malignant tumor. No che-

The work of Katherine M. Aferiat's 1988 unpublished professional paper *Application of Beck's Cognitive Theory of Depression to Nursing Practice* is acknowledged, particularly in the area of planning nursing actions.

motherapy or radiation was considered necessary because her physician believed the surgery was effective in curing her malignancy.

Mrs. Moon is the mother of three children, all in their early twenties. She has always been considered a pessimist, but after having surgery she sees herself as unattractive to her husband, an inadequate mother, and a social misfit. She avoids contact with others, seeing herself as an undesirable companion to others because of her cancer.

She verbalizes that others are afraid they will "catch" cancer from her and, thus, they avoid her. She says, "No one would want to have anything to do with a person with cancer." She lives alone with her husband, who works long and irregular hours. Her major social outlet has been through her church, but she has not attended any church activities since her surgery. She is having difficulty sleeping, has had bouts of crying, and her appetite has decreased. She claims, "My life is over. I don't enjoy anything anymore. Nothing gives me pleasure."

She has not resumed her usual social activities with her husband, saying, "My husband isn't interested in me anymore since I am no longer a real woman." She has rejected making holiday plans with her children saying, "My children don't need me." Her husband viewed her isolation from her family someone differently, saying, "She doesn't seem to want to have anything to do with her family and our old friends."

She presents herself to the clinic nurse, Mrs. Jones, without makeup and wearing an outdated skirt and blouse. She had formally been fashionably dressed. When Mrs. Jones asked her which of her symptoms concerned her the most, Mrs. Moon responded, tearfully, "My lack of contact with my family and my friends makes me feel that getting up in the morning is meaningless".

PATTERNING OF CUES FROM CLIENT CASE

The nurse initiates the strategy for providing theory-directed nursing practice for the Moon case. First she identifies the discrepancies in the case between the way the situation is and the way the situation should be. A discrepancy exists between Mrs. Moon's perception that her illness is hopeless and the medical probability that she is cured, between her usual social activities and her current social isolation, and between her former well-groomed appearance and her current disheveled appearance. Using the reasoning process of induction, Mrs. Jones identifies the following cues: difficulty sleeping, loss of appetite, bouts of crying, social isolation, decreased attention to appearance, unrealistic perception of the seriousness of her illness, decreased motivation to do anything, the perception that nothing gives her pleasure, perception that her husband and children do not need her anymore, and the belief that others avoid her because she has cancer.

The nurse recognizes a pattern of depression. Organizing these cues into a pattern, Mrs. Jones realizes she is faced with the problem of how to help Mrs. Moon change her view of herself as ill, unwanted, and miserable (depressed) to no longer ill, wanted, and reasonably content with her life (not depressed). The next step in the strategy for theory-directed nursing is the linking of the identified pattern from the case data to the theories stored in long-term memory.

SELECTED RELEVANT THEORIES

A number of theories could be used in providing care for Mrs. Moon. Three theories will be considered in order to illustrate that various theories provide different explanations for Mrs. Moon's behavior, leading to different etiologies for the nursing diagnoses and, therefore, different nursing interventions. The theories considered are psychoanalytic theory (Freud, 1957), behavioral theory (Lewinsohn, 1974), and cognitive theory of depression (Beck, 1976; Beck et al., 1979; Wright & Beck, 1983).

Freud's Intrapsychic Psychoanalytic Theory

One theory that might be considered for this case situation is the psychoanalytic theory of Freud (1957). This theory views depression as the turning inward of the aggressive instinct. The anger is not expressed toward the object of anger but displaced onto the self. Freud argued that the client is unable to recognize the anger as one of the components of his feelings toward an object.

The nursing diagnosis generated from this theory is "depression related to anger misdirected at self." Nursing interventions would be focused on changing the object on which Mrs. Moon directs her anger.

Lewinsohn's Behavioral Theory

Another theory that might be considered for this case situation would be Lewinsohn's (1974) behavioral theory. According to this theory, a low rate of reinforcement predisposes the individual to depression. The individual may fail to initiate the appropriate responses to receive positive reinforcements. In addition the environment may fail to provide the reinforcement because the depressed person's behavior may be perceived as depressing and negative.

The nursing diagnosis generated from this theory is "depression related to reinforcement deprivation." Interventions would be directed toward increasing the frequency and variety of pleasure-producing activities. Social skills training would also be used by the nurse to maximize the reinforcement obtained from others.

Beck's Cognitive Theory

Beck (1976) views cognition as the primary determinant of mood and behavior. He associates depression with an irrational thinking style. He believes that this irrational thinking style needs to be modified so that the thinking is more positive and realistic. Depressed people perceive themselves as losers; intervention is designed to make depressed people perceive themselves more like winners.

Beck's theory provides an explanation for why Mrs. Moon has generally considered herself a loser (distorted thinking) and why she is currently depressed (disturbed emotion). Beck's theory has been used effectively with medically ill populations (Dreyfus, 1988). In addition Beck's theory encompasses interventions that can be readily applied in the ambulatory setting. For these reasons it has been selected for illustration in this client situation.

DESCRIPTION OF BECK'S COGNITIVE THEORY OF DEPRESSION

Cognitive theories, in general, view distorted cognition (thinking) as the cause of maladaptive affect and behavior. Cognitive learning theory focuses on interventions aimed at cognitive restructuring. Beck's cognitive theory views depression as essentially a disorder of thinking rather than affect. Depression results primarily from the ways individuals evaluate their experiences rather than from unpleasant experiences as such.

The reader is reminded that the description of Beck's theory is brief because of space restrictions. It is assumed that a reader who wishes to utilize Beck's theory will seek out additional sources (especially primary sources) that describe the theory. Major primary sources of the theory include publications by Beck and others (Beck, 1976; Beck et al., 1979; Kovacs & Beck, 1978; and Wright & Beck, 1983). Burns (1980) published an excellent book in which Beck's theory is presented as a self-help guide. Secondary sources, in which Beck's theory is presented in the context of nursing, include Helm (1984), Hughes (1991), Dreyfus (1988), Manderino and Bzdek (1986), and Roberts (1989).

Beck's theory is complex and addresses multiple concepts. The author of this chapter, therefore, has selected those concepts she believes to be most pertinent to the case presentation. These selected concepts are named, theoretically defined, with clinical examples of the selected concepts identified and major relational statements presented.

Major Concepts

Cognition refers to both the content of thought and the processes involved in thinking. The content of thought describes what is being thought. The process of thought describes how knowledge is acquired and how beliefs are formed. Beck's theory focuses on three major concepts: cognitive triad, schemas, and cognitive errors. Table 4.1 presents a summary list of these three major concepts and their selected subconcepts. The three major concepts are presented and classified as content or process.

Theoretical Definitions of Major Concepts

Content of Cognition—Negative Cognitive Triad

One of the three major concepts focuses on the content of cognition—the negative cognitive triad. Beck's negative cognitive triad consists of three major cognitive patterns that determine:

Table 4.1   Major Concepts of Beck's Cognitive Theory of Depression

Content of Cognition—Negative Cognitive Triad
  Negative View of Self
  Negative View of Present
  Negative View of Future
Process of Cognition
  Schemas (Cognitive Structures)
  Faulty Information Processing (Cognitive Errors)
    Arbitrary inference
    Selective abstraction
    Overgeneralization
    Magnification and minimization
    Personalization
    Absolutistic, dichotomous thinking
    Disqualifying the positive
    Emotional reasoning
    Should statements
    Labeling and mislabeling

(1) Negative view of self—how a person regards self
(2) Negative view of present—how a person regards the present
(3) Negative view of future—how a person regards the future

The person's depressed affect is precipitated by the content of these negative, habitual, automatic thoughts.

Process Involved in Cognition

The other two major concepts are categorized as the processes associated in thinking: schemas (cognitive structures) and faulty information processing (cognitive errors).

Schemas (Cognitive Structures). Cognitive structures (schemas) represent relatively enduring structures that function like a template. The cognitive structures determine how information is screened, coded, categorized, and evaluated. Schemas are organized representations of prior experience. When a person is confronted with a particular situation, a schema is activated that is relevant to the situation. Schemas account for the idiosyncratic meaning people ascribe to their experiences. Maladaptive schemas are conclusions about cause and effect relationships that are based on false information or inadequate testing. The schema commonly associated with depression is negative value judgments.

Cognitive Errors (Faulty Information Processing). Cognitive errors occur when a maladaptive underlying schema is activated by an event. Beck described six cognitive errors: arbitrary inference, selective abstraction, over-generalization, magnification (catastrophizing) and minimization, personalization, and dichotomous thinking. Burns (1980), a colleague of Beck's, identified four additional cognitive errors: disqualifying the positive, emotional reasoning, should statements, and labeling and mislabeling. These ten cognitive errors are defined as follows:

1. *Arbitrary inference* ". . . refers to the process of drawing a specific conclusion in the absence of evidence to support the conclusion or when the evidence is contrary to the conclusion" (Beck et al., p. 14). In depression, arbitrary inference involves the drawing of negative conclusions in the absence of supporting data. Burns (1980) further classified arbitrary inference into two types: mind reading (making assumptions and arbitrary conclusions about how someone else feels or thinks without checking the data); the fortune telling error (predicting a negative outcome in the future and convincing yourself it is already a fact).

2. *Selective abstraction* refers to the ". . . focusing on a detail taken out of context, ignoring other more salient features of the situation and conceptualizing the whole experience on the basis of this fragment" (Beck et al., 1979, p. 14). Burns (1980) called this concept mental filter.

3. *Overgeneralization* ". . . refers to the pattern of drawing a general rule or conclusion on the basis of one or more isolated incidents and applying the concept across the board to related and unrelated situations" (Beck et al., 1979, p. 14).

4. *Magnification and minimization* refers to ". . . errors in evaluating the significance or magnitude of an event that are so gross as to constitute a distortion (Beck et al., 1979, p. 14). This process involves overestimating the importance of some events (usually failures) and downplaying others (usually successes). Burn's further described this concept as catastrophizing and "binocular trick." Catastrophizing is magnifying the potential importance or consequences of one small problem or mistake.

5. *Personalization* refers to the tendency to relate external events to self when there is no basis for making such a connection (Beck et al., 1979, p. 14). This concept involves blaming oneself for events that one did not have complete control over and using this belief to reinforce one's lack of self-worth.

6. *Absolutistic, dichotomous thinking* refers to the tendency to place all experiences in one of two opposite categories; the depressed person selects the extreme negative category (Beck et al., 1979, p. 14). Burns refers to this concept as all-or-nothing thinking.
7. *Disqualifying the positive* is defined as rejecting all positive experiences as meaningless (Burns, 1980).
8. *Emotional reasoning* is defined as assuming that negative feelings are representative of the way things really are. If you feel hopeless, then your problems must be impossible to solve (Burns, 1980).
9. *Should statements* are defined as both motivating oneself by "shoulds," which induces guilt, and directing "should" toward others, which results in anger and frustration (Burns, 1980). "Shoulds" are based on a personal set of inflexible rules for how people should behave and how life should be.
10. *Labeling and mislabeling* are an extreme form of overgeneralization. Labeling involves the labeling of behavior rather than the describing of behavior. "Mislabeling involves describing an event with language that is highly colored and emotionally loaded" (Burns, 1980, p. 41).

Examples of Concepts Relevant to Clinical Practice

Clinical examples for the concepts classified under content of thought (negative cognitive triad), and process of thought (schemas and cognitive errors) are presented.

Terry Smith, a senior nursing student, was criticized by Dr. Mary Shawn, her clinical instructor, for her performance on the first day of her senior leadership clinical assignment. Terry, whom the faculty viewed as an unusually competent and conscientious student, concluded "I am worthless" (negative view of self, cognitive distortion of labeling); "Now I'm a total failure" (negative view of present, cognitive distortion of overgeneralization); I'll never be a successful nurse" (negative view of future, cognitive distortion of fortune telling, overgeneralization). Terry's thoughts reveal the following schema. If people criticize me, I must be a bad person. In order to be happy I have to be successful in whatever I do.

Terry continued to berate herself. "I have let down my family" (cognitive error of arbitrary inference, mind reading, and magnification). "The faculty will never respect me again" (mind reading).

After the clinical instructor told Terry what behaviors were found lacking, she praised Terry for the effective behaviors she had performed that day. Terry heard only the negative criticisms (cognitive error of selective abstraction and mental filter). Her peers related how difficult they had also found their first experience. Terry, however, perceived that her poor performance jeopardized both the patients, hospital, and her school's future (personalization). Terry expected that she should (should statement) always be evaluated as exceptional in her nursing performance, that she should never make a mistake, and that a nurse who makes a mistake is a failure (labeling).

Terry's cognitions succeeded in making her feel thoroughly miserable. Because she felt so miserable, she refused to attend the play that the senior class had scheduled that evening. She spent the evening in the dormitory alone and continued to feel depressed and think about her personal failure. She dreaded going on the unit in the morning and considered calling in sick. She cried and had a sleepless night. She sought out her peers and said, "I can't stand it" (magnification). "I never do anything right" (overgeneralization). "I work hard but all Dr. Shawn does is criticize. She is a jerk" (mislabeling)!

Major Relational Statements

The major relational statements of the theory that link the major concepts with the concept of depression and form the basis for intervention follow.

1. Cognitions can determine affect, such as depression.
2. Affect and behavior are largely determined by the way in which the individual structures the world (schema, cognitive structure).
3. The signs and symptoms of the depressive syndrome are consequences of the activation of negative cognitive patterns.
4. Faulty information processing in the thinking of the depressed person maintains the person's belief in the validity of his or her negative concepts despite the presence of contradictory evidence.
5. Cognitive structures and faulty information processing can be modified.

IMPLICATIONS OF BECK'S THEORY OF DEPRESSION FOR CLINICAL PRACTICE

This section presents the use of Beck's theory of depression in nursing practice. Factors to be assessed, methods of assessing, theory-specific diagnoses, care planning, and evaluation of care are presented.

Factors to be Assessed and Methods of Assessing

The factors to be assessed include the level of suicidal ideation, the level of hopelessness, the target symptoms of depression, and the content and process of thought. Each of these factors are addressed.

Level of Suicidal Ideation

Because suicidal wishes are a prevalent and potentially lethal problem in depressed patients, the degree of suicidal intentions is assessed. The Scale for Suicide Ideation (Beck et al., 1979) can be utilized to assess suicide ideation in terms of attitudes towards living and dying, suicide ideation/wish, characteristics of a contemplated attempt, preparation for an attempt, and previous history of attempts.

Level of Hopelessness

Beck et al. (1979) advocate that the patient's sense of hopelessness be assessed in the first interview. Beck, Weisman, Lester, and Trexler (1974) developed a Hopelessness Scale for use in indirectly assessing the degree of suicide risk. A high score on this scale is a sign of high suicidal intent and is a better predictor of suicidal intent than depression (Beck, Kovacs, & Weisman, 1975).

Target Symptoms of Depression

Each depressed person reports a particular set of symptoms or problems that represent the most annoying aspect of the disorder. Beck referred to these as target symptoms. The five target symptom areas are: affective symptoms, motivational symptoms, cognitive symptoms, behavioral symptoms, and physiological or vegetative symptoms. According to Beck, the nurse and patient would decide which of the target symptoms should be addressed on the basis of which are the most distressing to the patient, and which are most amenable to therapeutic intervention.

Content and Process of Thought

A number of instruments that can be utilized in assessing the content and process of thought have been generated. Two will be described here: Beck's Depression Inventory (BDI) and the General Cognitive Error Questionnaire.

Beck's Depression Inventory. Beck's Depression Inventory (Beck, 1976, Beck et al., 1979) can be used to assess the severity of the depression, determine the existence of certain target symptoms such as suicidal wishes, and the individual's negative thoughts. The BDI is a 21-item self-administered questionnaire. Each item contains four choices of responses rated from 0 to 3. The total score is obtained by adding up the score for each item. The higher the score, the more severe the depression. Burns (1980) asserted that a score of 10 or below could be considered within normal limits; a score over 20 indicates a clinical depression.

The General Cognitive Error Questionnaire. The General Cognitive Error Questionnaire (LeFebvre, 1981) assesses the level of distortion of four cognitive errors: catastrophizing, overgeneralization, personalization, and selective abstraction. The questionnaire is composed of 24 short vignettes. Each vignette is followed by a dysphoric cognition that reflects a cognitive error. Subjects are asked to rate how similar the cognition is to how they would think in a similar situation. This rating is made up of a 5-point scale ranging from "almost exactly like I would think" to "not all like I would think." The content of the vignettes is evenly divided across work, family/ home, and recreation activities. Values from 0 to 4 are assigned to the response choices. The scores for an individual cognitive error are the total of the numerical equivalents of the response choices selected on the items reflecting that cognitive error. Possible scores range from 0 to 24. A high score indicates a high degree of that specific cognitive error.

Schemas

Schemas are also assessed as they "may be latent but can be activated by specific circumstances which are analogous to experiences initially responsible for embedding the negative attitude" (Beck et al., 1979, p. 16). "The precipitants of depression revolve around a perceived or actual loss . . ." (Beck et al., 1979, p. 24). Beck believed that the individual remains vulnerable to future depressions unless the schemas are identified and changed. Schemas are inferred from the dysfunctional cognitions. For example, depression ". . . may be triggered by a physical abnormality or disease that activates a person's latent belief that he is destined for a life of suffering" (Beck et al., 1979, p. 16).

Theory-Specific Diagnoses

A generic nursing diagnosis that is generated from Beck's theory is depression related to distortions in cognitive thinking. A more specific nursing diagnosis reflecting the generic one is recommended because it may be more helpful in generating the nursing care plan.

Response Component

Beck et al. (1979) asserted that "in the moderately to severely depressed patient, the focus of the therapeutic intervention should be at the target symptom level" (p. 96). The patient is provided with symptom relief by translating the patient's symptoms into solvable problems. Target symptoms are perceived as solvable problems. Thus, in addition to identifying depression in the response component of the nursing diagnosis, the target symptoms of depression could be used in identifying more specific response components. Potential specific response components are:

Affective Target Symptoms
Sadness
Loss of gratification
Apathy
Loss of feelings and affection toward others
Loss of mirth responses
Motivational Target Symptoms
Wish to escape from life (often by suicide)
Wish to avoid problems or even everyday activities
Cognitive Target Symptoms
Difficulty in concentrating
Problems in attention span
Difficulties in memory
Behavioral Target Symptoms
Passivity
Withdrawal from others
Motor retardation

Agitation
Physiological or Vegetative Target Symptoms
Sleep disturbance (either increased or decreased)
Appetite disturbance (either increased or decreased)

Etiology Component

Beck recognizes the etiology of depression as multiple. However, he believes that cognitive distortions play a major role in the etiology of depression. The depressed person fails to distinguish between internal mental processes and the outside world that stimulates them. The depressed person possesses insufficient knowledge regarding procedures for acquiring accurate knowledge.

The ten types of cognitive errors (distortions) thus make up a typology of etiology components for generating the nursing diagnosis statement. Some examples of etiologies are:

1. Drawing of negative conclusions in the absence of supporting data (arbitrary inference)
2. Making conclusions about how others feel or think without checking with them (mind reading)
3. Predicting a negative outcome and believing the prediction is a fact (the fortune telling trick)
4. Focusing on negative details of a situation (selective abstraction, mental filter)
5. Drawing conclusions on the basis of isolated data or irrelevant data (overgeneralization)
6. Over-estimating failure and downplaying successes (magnification and minimization)
7. Magnifying the potential consequences (catastrophizing)
8. Blaming self for events one has no control over (personalization)
9. Placing all experience in a negative light (absolutistic, dichotomous thinking)
10. Rejecting positive experiences (disqualifying the positive)
11. Assuming that negative feelings are the way things really are (emotional reasoning)
12. Trying to live by a set of inflexible rules (should statements)
13. Equating oneself or others with what one does (labeling and mislabeling)

Sample Nursing Diagnoses

A selection from the response and etiology examples, generated from Beck's theory, were used to generate the following examples of nursing diagnoses.

1. *Potential for suicide (depression—motivational target symptom) related to labeling self as hopeless (labeling).* Suicidal intent is associated more strongly with the degree of hopelessness than with the intensity of depression (Beck, 1976).
2. *Loss of gratification in activities of daily living (depression—affective target symptom) related to trying to live with a set of inflexible rules (should statements).* When the reality of behavior falls short of standards, the shoulds and shouldn'ts create self-blaming, shame, and guilt (Burns, 1980).
3. *Withdrawal from others (depression—behavioral target symptom) related to making conclusions about how others feel or think without checking with them (mind reading).* Depressed persons have difficulty in assessing the accuracy of feedback (Wright & Beck, 1983).
4. *Decreased ability to sleep (depression—physiological target symptom) related to focusing on negative details of a situation (selective abstraction).* Depressed subjects have been found to overestimate the amount of negative feedback and underestimate the amount of positive feedback they receive (Wright & Beck, 1983).
5. *Difficulty concentrating on school assignments (depression—cognitive target symptom) related to predicting a negative outcome and believing the prediction is a fact (the fortune telling trick).* "Apathy and low energy may result from the patient's belief that he is doomed to failure in all efforts" (Beck et al., 1979, p. 12). The depressed patient ". . . is completely preoccupied with preservative, repetitive negative thoughts and may find it enormously difficult to concentrate on external stimuli . . ." (Beck et al., 1979, p. 13).

Care Plan

Because depression consists of affective, motivational, cognitive, behavioral, and physiological components, the nurse can concentrate on any one or a combination of these components to induce a change in the total syndrome of depression. Each of the components has a reciprocal relationship with the other components, and therefore, improvement in one major problem area generally spreads into the others.

Intervention consists of breaking up the complex phenomenon of depression into component problems (client response and etiology), selecting the specific problems (nursing diagnosis) to be addressed in a given case, and then determining what types of therapeutic interventions would be appropriate (based on etiology component). Interventions consist of behavioral reactivation by identifying and correcting habitual negative appraisals. Interventions include both behavioral and cognitive strategies.

Behavioral Strategies

If the depression is severe, it is necessary to start first with behavioral strategies to reactivate the client. These strategies consist of activity schedules, mastery and pleasure schedules, and graded task assignments.

The activity schedule consists of a schedule of activities for the day. It is used as a motivational tool in overcoming lethargy and preoccupation with depressive ideas.

A mastery and pleasure schedule consists of the person keeping an account of daily activities. The client places an "M" on activities that have been mastered; a "P" is placed on activities that gave pleasure. This strategy is designed to help the client perceive successes and to focus on the pleasurable aspects of life, which they have failed to perceive as such in the past.

Graded task assignments consist of breaking up large tasks into small manageable steps. It is designed to permit the client to experience success first in simple tasks and then in more complex tasks.

Cognitive Strategies

Strategies designed to identify and correct habitual negative appraisals include: patient self-monitoring, hypothesis testing, problem solving, patient self-monitoring of dysfunctional thoughts and alternative rational interpretations, and basic assumption modification. Clients are provided with the rationale for the nursing interventions, that is, the low mood, behavioral disruption, lack of motivation, and vegetative symptoms are the consequences of distorted negative thinking (Helm, 1984). The client is taught to differentiate between belief and fact by collecting evidence that would support or disconfirm negative perceptions and beliefs.

Self-monitoring consists of the client observing and recording cognitions and accompanying affect. This is designed to help differentiate thoughts from feelings.

Hypothesis testing consists of the nurse and the client examining the client's cognitions. This involves careful questioning regarding the validity of the appraisals and what implications these appraisals have for the past, present, and future.

Problem solving involves the nurse and the client engaging in realistic problem solving by looking for plausible solutions to real life situations.

A daily record of dysfunctional thoughts consists of having the client write down situations that bring on depressed moods, the degree of emotion experienced in the situation, the automatic thought associated with the emotion, the cognitive distortion, the rational response, and the outcome emotion.

Basic assumption modification is achieved through the client and the nurse inferring basic cognitive themes or premises (schemas) from the patient's interpretation of daily events.

Implementation of the Care Plan

During the implementation of the plan of care, the patient and nurse change the plan when they believe it is appropriate. The patient takes an active role in implementing and modifying the plan.

Evaluation of the Care Plan

The care plan evaluation is ongoing. Both the patient and the nurse participate in the evaluation. The behavior used as the response component is the behavior the patient has claimed is the most problematic. As that behavior becomes less problematic, a favorable product outcome evaluation occurs. As the errors in thinking become less automatic and the patient shows improvement in obtaining the needed information from the environment in order to form rational cognitions, a favorable process evaluation occurs.

THEORY-DIRECTED NURSING CARE FOR MRS. MOON

Beck's cognitive theory of depression is applied to Mrs. Moon's case. Each of the five steps of the nursing process is illustrated.

Assessing

The assessment data are organized under the indicators of depression (target symptoms, hopelessness, suicidal ideation) and the content and process of thought. Mrs. Moon received a score of 26 on the depression inventory, indicating that she is clinically moderately depressed. Upon questioning, she denied any active suicidal ideation. On question number 9 of the BDI, she checked "I don't have any thoughts about killing myself." Her responses are classified into the five target symptoms described by Beck.

1. Affective symptoms
   I don't enjoy anything anymore; nothing gives me pleasure
   Crying bouts
2. Motivational symptoms
   Loss of interest in her personal appearance
   Avoidance of social activities
3. Cognitive symptoms
   View that illness is overwhelming
4. Behavioral symptoms
   Withdrawal from others
   "My lack of contact with my family and my friends makes me feel that getting up in the morning is meaningless"
5. Physiological or vegetative symptoms
   Difficulty sleeping
   Decrease in appetite

Mrs. Moon revealed the following cognitive distortions:

1. Arbitrary inference (mind reading): No one would want to be around someone with cancer. My husband doesn't view me as a real woman anymore. My children don't need me.
2. Magnification: My condition is hopeless.
3. Should: Real women should have a uterus.

4. Overgeneralization: Because I got cancer, my life is over.
5. Labeling: I am hopeless.
6. Emotional reasoning: Since I feel hopeless, my cancer is hopeless.
7. Selective abstraction: Mrs. Moon "heard" that she had cancer; she did not "hear" that surgery had removed the cancer.

The pattern of the cognitive distortions suggests that Mrs. Moon has an underlying schema that she is destined for a life of suffering.

Diagnosing

Because depression is a phenomena characterized by a number of target symptoms, more than one nursing diagnosis would be generated for Mrs. Moon. Only one diagnosis, however, is illustrated in this paper. The following diagnosis was formulated based on the data presented in the clinical case and the target symptom Mrs. Moon believed was the most problematic.

Social Isolation (Depression—Behavioral Target Symptom) Related to Belief that Others do not Wish to be Around Someone with Cancer (Arbitrary Inference)

The subjective and objective data that support the diagnosis are presented.

Response: social isolation (depression—behavioral target symptom)

Subjective Data	**Objective Data**
"My wife doesn't seem to want to have anything to do with her family or our old friends."	No longer attending church activities or carrying out activities with husband and children.
"My lack of contact with my family and my friends makes me feel that getting up in the morning is meaningless".	

Etiology: Belief that others do not wish to be around someone who has cancer (arbitrary inference)

Subjective Data   **Objective Data**
"No one would want to have any-   No objective data presented.
thing to do with a person with can-
cer."

Planning

Based on the response component of the nursing diagnosis, *social isolation,*
goals and predicted outcomes have been formulated.

Goal: Mrs. Moon will resume her church activities and her activities with her
husband and children.

Predicted Outcomes:

1. Mrs. Moon will attend one church activity within the next month.
2. Mrs. Moon will participate in at least one event with each member of
   her family—husband, son, and daughter—within the next month.
3. Mrs. Moon will participate in an event with all of her family within 5
   weeks.
4. Mrs. Moon will attend a major church social event within 6 weeks.

Based on the etiology component of the nursing diagnosis, *belief that others
do not want to be around someone with cancer*, the nursing interventions and
nursing actions are planned.

Nursing Interventions:
Teach the client to differentiate between belief and fact by assisting her to put
her perception that others don't want to be around a person who has cancer to
empirical test.

Nursing Actions   **Rationale**
1. Set an agenda for each meeting   ". . . since depressed people have an
   with Mrs. Moon and during the   impairment in learning and memory
   meeting ascertain that the agen-   function, the therapy should be high-
   da is appropriate.   ly structured and should encourage
                                       clear communication . . ." (Wright
                                       & Beck, 1983, p. 1122).

2. Help Mrs. Moon identify the basis of her beliefs regarding how others feel about being around people with cancer.

"Direct questioning is the most frequent technique used to elicit automatic thoughts and distorted beliefs" (Wright & Beck, 1983, p. 1122).

3. Ask Mrs. Moon to read chapter 1 through 3 in *Feeling Good* by David Burns and discuss it with the nurse.

This book "helps the patient to learn about cognitive therapy treatment procedures" (Wright & Beck, 1983, p. 1122).

"Homework assignments are also used to augment the learning process" (Wright & Beck, 1983, p. 1122).

4. Have Mrs. Moon write down examples of thinking errors.

Labeling and categorizing automatic thoughts can provide some objectivity and distancing (Beck, 1976).

5. Ask Mrs. Moon to consider her choice of the automatic thought that others don't want to be around her as an hypothesis.

"The cognitive therapist asks the client to suspend temporarily his conviction that the thought is unquestionably true and instead to treat it as an hypothesis to be tested" (Young, 1982, p. 386).

"Automatic thoughts are conscious and can be retrieved" (Wright & Beck, 1983, p. 1120).

6. Have Mrs. Moon write down the evidence for and against the thought.

"The therapist and client collaborate in assembling evidence that supports and contradicts the thought, in evaluating this evidence, and in drawing conclusions" (Young, 1982, p. 386).

7. Encourage Mr. Moon to decide the outcome of the evidence.

"Clients discover the inconsistencies for themselves instead of having them pointed out" (Young, 1982, 386).

8 Work with Mrs. Moon in devising rational responses to the negative thought if there is no evidence for the thought.

"Usually the painful emotional state diminishes as the patient is able to disprove negatively distorted thinking" (Wright & Beck, 1983, p. 1123).

9. If the evidence is inconclusive, collaborate with Mrs. Moon in setting up an experiment to test the hypothesis.

"A powerful method with which to investigate the validity of a specific assumption consists of designing an experiment or task to test the assumption empirically" (Beck et al., 1979, p. 56).

10. If the negative thought is true, assist Mrs. Moon in problem solving.

"Patient and therapist engage in realistic problem solving, looking for plausible solutions to real life problems" (Helm, 1984, p. 104).

11. Explore underlying assumptions that fuel Mrs. Moon's negative thinking.

Changing the patient's erroneous or dysfunctional assumptions has a direct effect upon the patient's ability to avoid future depressions (Beck et al., 1979).

Implementing

The nurse performed the planned nursing actions to facilitate the achievement of the client goal and predicted outcomes. The nurse met with Mrs. Moon for one hour two times a week for 5 weeks. They had originally planned to meet for 6 weeks, but Mrs. Moon and her family went away on a week's vacation so the sixth meeting did not take place.

The nurse explained the rationale behind cognitive therapy and asked Mrs. Moon to read the first three chapters in Burn's book *Feeling Good*. Mrs. Moon read only the first chapter the first week it was assigned. The nurse asked Mrs. Moon the reason for not completing the assignment and Mrs. Moon, said, "I just thought it wouldn't really help. My situation is hopeless." The nurse used this as an example of how negative thinking can perpetuate depressed feelings. Mrs. Moon completed her reading the following week and verbalized that she was beginning to understand her role in causing her feelings of rejection from others and her depression.

Mrs. Moon and the nurse mutually set the agenda for each meeting. On two occasions they changed the session agenda at midsession because one of them indicated that the agenda was not appropriate. The first time it was the nurse who questioned its appropriateness, the second time it was Mrs. Moon who questioned its appropriateness.

The nurse taught Mrs. Moon how to keep the Daily Record of Dysfunctional Thoughts by showing her an example and helping her write the first day's record. The nurse worked with Mrs. Moon in testing out the negative thought that other people do not want to be around people with cancer. Mrs. Moon was encouraged to test this thought using evidence for and evidence against. She concluded that only one of her acquaintances admitted to a fear of being around a person with cancer. She found that when she made efforts to be around other people, they generally accepted and welcomed her presence in much the same manner as they had before her illness.

Evaluating

Both product and process outcome evaluations are conducted.

Product Evaluation (Extent That Goals and Predicted Outcomes Were Met).

1. Mrs. Moon attended her Sunday School class party during the second week of treatment. She had planned to leave early but was enjoying herself so much, she remained until the party ended.
2. Mrs. Moon had dinner with her husband and daughter during the third week of treatment.
3. Mrs. Moon attended her son's baseball game during the fourth week of treatment.
4. Mrs. Moon, her husband, daughter, and son went to a restaurant for dinner and attended a play during the fifth week of treatment.
5. Mrs. Moon planned to attend the mother-daughter banquet at her church; her daughter was not able to attend. She attended the banquet with her neighbor and her neighbor's daughter. She said that she understood that her daughter's social conflicts prevented her from attending and it was not that she did not wish to spend time with her mother.

Process Evaluation

Nurse Focus (extent that planned nursing interventions and nursing actions were implemented).

1. The nurse met with Mrs. Moon for five of the planned six sessions.
2. An agenda was set for each meeting and it was modified on two

occasions, once at the request of the nurse and once at the request of Mrs. Moon.

3. The nurse asked Mrs. Moon to read the relevant chapters in Burns' book.

4. The nurse requested that Mrs. Moon write down examples of thinking errors, to reconsider her choice of an automatic thought as an hypothesis, and to write down the evidence for and against the thought.

Client Focus (extent that etiology component of the nursing diagnosis statement was modified).

Mrs. Moon checked her belief that others did not want to be around a person with cancer. She determined that many of her friends not only did not have this belief but had experienced cancer themselves.

SUMMARY

This section described and applied Beck's Cognitive Theory of Depression, in the context of the nursing process, to a client who experienced a diagnosis of cancer. The application of Beck's theory demonstrates that clients can modify the affect of depression by changing the way they think about the events that happen to them.

REFERENCES

Beck, A. T. (1976). *Cognitive therapy and emotional disorders.* New York: International Universities Press.

Beck, A. T., Kovacs, M., & Weismann, A. (1975). Hopelessness and suicidal behavior: An overview. *Journal of the American Medical Association, 234,* 1146–1149.

Beck, A. T., Rush, A. J., Shaw, B. G., & Emery, G. (1979). *Cognitive therapy of depression.* New York: Guilford.

Beck, A. T., Weisman, A., Lester, D., & Trexler, L. (1974). The measurement of pessimism: The Hopelessness Scale. *Journal of Consulting and Clinical Psychology, 42,* 861–865.

Burns, D. D. (1980). *Feeling good: The new mood therapy.* New York: William Morrow.

Campbell, L. (1987). Hopelessness. *Journal of Psychosocial Nursing, 25*(2), 18–22.

Dreyfus, J. K. (1988). The treatment of depression in an ambulatory care setting. *Nurse Practitioner, 13*(7), 14–33.

Freud, S. (1957). Mourning and melancholia. In J. Strachey & A. Tyson (Translators) *The complete works of Sigmund Freud*, Vol. 14. London: The Hogarth Press, Ltd.

Helm, S. B. (1984). Nursing care of the depressed patient: Cognitive approach. *Perspectives in Psychiatric Care, 22*, 100–107.

Hughes, C. P. (1991). Community psychiatric nursing and the depressed elderly: A case for using cognitive therapy. *Journal of Advanced Nursing, 16*, 565–572.

Kovacs, M., & Beck, A. T. (1978). Maladaptive cognitive structures in depression. *The American Journal of Psychiatry, 135*, 525–533.

Krantz, S., & Hammen, C. (1979). Assessment of cognitive bias in depression. *Journal of Abnormal Psychology, 88*, 611–619.

LeFebvre, M. F. (1981). Cognitive distortion and cognitive errors in depressed psychiatric and low back pain patients. *Journal of Consulting and Clinical Psychology, 49*, 517–525.

Lewinsohn, P. M. (1974). A behavioral approach to depression. In R. J. Friedman & M. Katz (Eds.) *The psychology of depression: Contemporary theory and research* (pp. 157–178). New York: Winston-Wiley.

Manderino, M. A., & Bzdek, V. M. (1986). Mobilizing depressed clients. *Journal of Psychosocial Nursing, 24*(5), 23–28.

Maurer, F. A. (1986). Acute depression: Treatment and nursing strategies for this affective disorder. *Nursing Clinics of North America, 21*, 413–427.

Roberts, S. L. (1989). Cognitive model of depression and the myocardial infarction patient. *Progress in Cardiovascular Nursing, 4*, 61–69.

Sideleau, B. F. (1987). Irrational beliefs and intervention. *Journal of Psychosocial Nursing, 25*(3), 18–24.

Wright, J. H, & Beck, A. T. (1983). Cognitive therapy of depression: Theory and practice. *Hospital and Community Psychiatry, 34*, 1119–1127.

Young, J. (1982). Loneliness, depression, and cognitive therapy: Theory and application. In L. Peplau & D. Perlman (Eds.) *Loneliness: A sourcebook of current theory, research and therapy* (pp. 379–404). New York: John Wiley & Sons.

Ziegler, S., Vaughan-Wrobel, B., & Erlen, J. (1986). *Nursing process, nursing diagnosis, nursing knowledge: Avenues to Autonomy*. Norwalk, CT: Appleton-Century-Crofts.

SUGGESTED READINGS

Freud, S. (1953–1974). In J. Strachey, (Ed.) *The standard edition of the complete psychological works of Sigmund Freud*. London: Hogarth Press.

Lewinsohn, P., & Amenson, C. Some relations between pleasant and unpleasant mood related activities and depression. *Journal Abnormal Psychology, 87*, 644.

Lewinsohn, P., Youngren, M., & Grosscup, S. (1979). Reinforcement and depression. In R. Depue (Ed.) *The psychobiology of the depressive disorders*. New York: Academic Press.

Chapter 5

Bowen's Family Theory

Wilda K. Arnold, Rose Nieswiadomy,
and Gail Walden Watson

Although nurses have long recognized the family as a focus for nursing, the major emphasis has frequently been placed on the individual rather than on the family. Family members share intense ties that must be considered when working with individuals or with families as a whole. Because of the complexity of the family system, theories to guide nursing practice with families are needed. Bowen's family theory is useful for nurses who are interacting with families in any setting.

CLIENT CASE

The Atkins family, composed of Richard (age 34), Alicia (age 22), and Patrick (age 3), moved to Detroit 3 months ago so that Richard might find better employment opportunities. Prior to the move, they had lived all their lives in New York. Richard quit his job in New York 9 months ago, forcing them to move in with Alicia's parents. Since moving to Detroit they have been living in a one-room efficiency apartment and Richard has found part-time employment in a labor pool. The income from this job does not cover the monthly bills; thus the couple has had to ask for financial assistance from their families. Richard uses their only car for work and job hunting, while Alicia and Patrick stay in the apartment all day.

Alicia was 6 months pregnant when they moved to Detroit, and last month she delivered a 5-pound son, who died 3 hours after birth because of respiratory distress. Following the infant's death, Alicia was often tearful and on several occasions refused to see Richard when he came to the hospital. She said, "He doesn't care about anything but himself. It's his fault the baby died." Alicia told the nurse, "We should never have come to Detroit." When the nurse attempted to discuss the relationship between the couple, Alicia quickly changed the subject and began to talk about the problems that Patrick was having.

A home health nurse began visiting the family after Alicia was discharged. She learned that Alicia continued to cry frequently, and the nurse determined that Alicia was depressed. According to Alicia, she and her husband had not been able to discuss the loss of the baby. When they did talk, they would begin arguing and yelling at each other, at which time Patrick would begin to cry. In addition, Patrick started to suck his thumb and say to his parents each night, "I want to sleep with you."

When a nurse from a support group visited the couple, Alicia seemed to be preoccupied with talking about Patrick and how concerned she was about his behaviors. Alicia stated, "I want to take Patrick and go home to New York. He would stop sucking his thumb and crying so much." Richard refused to discuss the subject saying, "My wife just doesn't understand me." At this point, Alicia said, "All Richard does is leave in the morning and come home smelling like liquor."

PATTERNING CUES FROM CLIENT CASE

The nurse examines the information that she has gathered from the family and determines that Patrick's behavior is a symptom of family problems. This decision is based upon the following cues:

1. Many changes have occurred for the family, including the move from New York.
2. Alicia and Richard have not dealt with the loss of their infant last month.
3. Richard blames Alicia for their problems, saying that she does not understand him, and Alicia blames Richard because she says he only thinks of himself.
4. Communication between the two results in arguments.

5. Patrick's behavior has regressed since his parents' relationship has become more overtly disturbed.

The nurse recognizes that in order for Patrick's behavior to change, the marital relationship will need to be improved. It will be important to work with the marital couple and help them to gain an understanding of what is occurring in their lives and how they can make the decision to change their beliefs and their behavior. The nurse will recall to active memory information about relevant theories that might be used in working with this family. Then one of these theories will be selected and the nursing process will be utilized based on the concepts and propositions of this theory.

SELECTED RELEVANT THEORIES

There are a number of family theories which could be used in working with the Atkins family. Three theories will be discussed to demonstrate how different theories can be applied in providing nursing care for this family. The three theories to be discussed are Minuchin's structural family theory, Satir's communication theory, and Bowen's family theory. Minuchin's and Satir's theories will be presented briefly. Then a more in-depth exploration and discussion of the use of Bowen's theory will be presented.

Minuchin's Structural Family Theory

According to Minuchin's (1974) theory, behavior is the result of the patterns of interaction among family members. Minuchin assumes that a person is not an isolate, but rather an interacting member of social groups. Thus, Minuchin is concerned with the family as a unit and not with each separate individual in the family.

Minuchin proposes that the family is a system in transition, the family moves through predictable stages of development, and the family has structure. If disturbances occur in any of these components, family dysfuction may occur. When faced with the need for change, family members may exhibit growth behaviors or respond with maladaptive behaviors.

Minuchin's theory includes several concepts, one of which is that of "boundaries." This concept concerns the family rules about who participates and how they participate in family interactions. In order for the family to function effectively, the boundaries must be well-defined. Minuchin discusses boundaries on a continuum. On one end of the continuum the boundaries are rigid (disengaged), while on the opposite end of the continuum boundaries are intertwined (enmeshed). Either of these extremes inhibit communication. In the middle of the continuum boundaries are clear-cut and communication is, thus, facilitated.

When working with families, the emphasis is not placed on the person with the problem, because everyone in the family has contributed to the problem. The emphasis is placed on changing patterns of actions to produce new feelings. Minuchin discusses teaching the family members new "scripts" to follow in their interactions with each other.

Minuchin encourages family members to talk to each other until he identifies the central issue; then he makes a determination of who is most involved with the issue. He examines such verbal communication patterns as interruptions and silences to try to determine what might be inhibiting the progress of the family discussion.

Minuchin often rearranges the setting, as if it were a stage. New seating assignments may be made. He encourages family members to be involved with each other in the discussion. For example, rather than saying "Why do you think your husband won't talk to you?" he might say, "Try to get your husband to talk to you right now."

A nursing diagnosis for the Atkins family, based on Minuchin's theory, is "Patrick's regressive behaviors related to enmeshed family boundaries." When using Minuchin's theory, the focus is placed on the family as a unit. The nurse assists the couple to learn new transactional behaviors and teaches them how to discuss issues as a family.

Satir's Communication Theory

Family therapy, according to Satir (1967) concerns communication among family members. Communication refers to all interactional behavior, including verbal and nonverbal behavior. It includes symbols and clues that people use in giving and receiving messages. Communication techniques that people use are fairly accurate indicators of interpersonal functioning. Thus, an analysis of an individual's or a family's communication patterns will help identify relationships between those communication patterns and dysfunctional behavior.

If an individual has not learned to communicate properly, this individual will be unable to perform the most important function of good communication, that of "checking out his or her perceptions to see whether they tally with the situation as it really is or with the intended meaning of another" (Satir, Stachowiak, & Taschman, 1983, p. 94). Problems in communication are closely related to an individual's self-image and self-esteem. For example, parents may not be good communication models and may send messages that devalue the child (Satir, 1967).

In discussing the family, Satir wrote that the marital relationship is the axis around which all other relationships in the family are developed. When the marital dyad is disturbed, there is a tendency toward dysfunctional parenting. The family member who is most affected by the disturbed marital relationship is called the "Identified Patient" (IP). This individual's symptoms are the result of the family imbalance and "are a message that he is distorting his own growth as a result of trying to alleviate and absorb his parents' pain" (Satir, 1967, p. 2).

Therapy is an effort to improve inadequate methods of communication. The focus is placed on correcting discrepancies in the family's communication process. The therapist teaches family members how to achieve clear communication by being a model of communication. The therapist is also a resource person who is an experienced and impartial observer capable of reporting accurately what he or she sees and hears. Rather than "joining" the family as some therapists do, Satir (1967) suggests that the therapist should remain outside the family and above the family's power struggles.

The nursing diagnosis generated from Satir's theory is "Patrick's regressive behaviors related to dysfunctional family communication." Nursing interventions focus on teaching the family functional communication techniques. The nurse models clear communication and points out to the family members when their communication patterns interfere with healthy functioning.

Bowen's Family Theory

Bowen's theory concerns the emotional functioning of the family. Bowen (1978) describes the family as a system and contends that pathology is a product of this system. When one member of the system changes, there will be changes in other members of the family. Bowen (1978) focuses on the interrelationships between the marital couple and on the extended families from generations past. The emotional system of each family member is tied to that of the other family members, both in the present and in the past. Therefore, the theory is called a systems theory as well as an intergenerational theory.

When a person can maintain a desirable degree of emotional separateness or individuality, problems are avoided. However, if members are too tied to each other emotionally, they become fused.

Bowen also discusses the need for differentiating between feelings and intellectual processes. He states, "the core of my theory has to do with the degree to which people distinguish between the feeling process and the intellectual process" (p. 355). When Bowen began conducting family research, he found that parents of schizophrenic patients might appear to be functioning well but were actually having difficulty distinguishing between the subjective feeling process and the objective thinking process. The more people are able to separate these two processes, the more they will be able to differentiate themselves from the family and become separate individuals. The inability to separate emotions from intellectual processes results in anxiety when stressful situations are encountered.

DESCRIPTION OF BOWEN'S FAMILY THEORY

The use of Bowen's theory in clinical cases will be discussed in this section of the chapter. The major concepts will be described and theoretically defined. Examples will be presented for the concepts that are most relevant to clinical practice with families. Finally, major relational statements from Bowen's theory will be identified. A thorough exploration of Bowen's theory is beyond the scope of this book. For more information about the theory the reader is referred to the references at the end of this chapter.

Major Concepts

According to Bowen (1978) humans have built-in mechanisms to deal with low levels of anxiety. When anxiety increases, tension develops. When a person's emotions and intellect are operating separately, that person will have more success in coping with tension. As emotions and intellect become fused, there is less integration of self. Differentiation of self is the cornerstone of Bowen's theory. The eight major concepts of Bowen's theory are presented in Table 5.1.

Theoretical Definitions of Major Concepts

Differentiation of Self

Differentiation of self has three elements, according to Bowen. (1978) The first of these, the inter-psychic element, describes the emotional "stuck-togetherness" in families. In mature families, individual members do not become involved in emotional fusion with each other. However, in undifferentiated families, members become emotionally fused with each other.

The second aspect of differentiation concerns the intra-psychic level of differentiation between emotions and intellect (Bowen, 1978). This differentiation occurs on a continuum ranging from low to high, and may vary from time to time. According to Bowen's theory, those on the high end of the continuum will be able to establish autonomous and independent lives from their families of origin. The differentiated person has intellectual and emotional systems that function separately. This individual makes decisions based on intellect and is apt to have fewer problems than those who are highly fused. Those with low levels of differentiation are dominated by emotions, are unable to differentiate facts from feelings, are relationship-oriented, and make decisions based on feelings.

Table 5.1 Major Concepts of Bowen's Family Theory

Differentiation of self
Triangles
Nuclear family emotional system
Family projection process
Emotional cutoff
Multigenerational transmission process
Sibling position
Societal regression

The third element of differentiation concerns the intra-psychic level of self-maturity. Bowen described the person as having a solid-self and a pseudo-self. He described the solid-self as "made up of clearly defined beliefs, opinions, convictions, and life principles" (p. 365). This solid-self is stable and can be changed from within the self, while the pseudo-self is acquired from others, is created by emotional pressures, is unstable, and can be changed by external forces.

Triangles

A triangle is "the smallest stable relationship system. A two-person system may be stable as long as it is calm, but when anxiety increases it immediately involves the most vulnerable other person to become a triangle" (Bowen, 1978, p. 373). The basic building block of any emotional system is the "triangle." Bowen (1971) observed that the "two-person system is an unstable system that immediately forms a series of interlocking triangles" (p. 394). The smaller two-person system may function satisfactorily until tension causes one or both of the individuals to feel discomfort. To relieve the tension, another person will be added to the system, forming a triangle. The twosome in the relationship will work to maintain the togetherness, while the third person (the outsider) will strive to form a togetherness with one of the twosome (Bowen, 1978). However, during times of stress the outside position is the most desirable.

Bowen (1978) further stated, "When it is not possible to shift forces in the triangle, one of the involved twosome triangles in a fourth, leaving the former third person aside for reinvolvement" (p. 373). Emotional forces of the original triangle will be repeated in the new triangle. When there are no new triangles available in the family, they will go outside the family system, seeking outsiders to help relieve the tension. Jones (1980) wrote that triangles are dysfunctional, preventing resolution of problems and further stated, "Repeated over time, triangling will become a chronic dysfunctional pattern, preventing resolution of differences in the marriage and making one or more of the threesome vulnerable to physical or emotional symptoms" (p. 48).

Nuclear Family Emotional System

The nuclear family emotional system is defined as "the patterns of emotional functioning in a family in a single generation. Certain basic patterns between the father, mother, and children are replicas of the past generations and will be repeated in the generations to follow" (Bowen, 1978, p. 376).

The concept of the nuclear family emotional system is concerned with a family's patterns of emotional functioning over the span of one generation. Persons select spouses with similar levels of differentiation which, in turn, influences the patterns of emotional functioning of the couple. Individuals with low levels of differentiation are more apt to develop problems (Bowen, 1978; Jones, 1980; Shealy, 1988). In writing about the levels of differentiation, Bowen (1978) noted, "the lower the level of differentiation, the more intense the emotional fusion of marriage" (p. 377). Fusion leads to anxiety, which must be dealt with in some way. The major ways families attempt to resolve this anxiety are through marital conflict, dysfunction of one spouse, and impairment in one or more of the children.

Family Projection Process

The family projection process is "the basic process by which parental problems are projected to children" (Bowen, 1971, p. 398). The family projection process involves the projection of parental conflict onto the child, which causes emotional impairment in the child. Bowen (1978) states that the process begins with an anxious mother. The child responds with anxiety to the mother's anxiety. The mother misperceives the behavior of the child as a problem in the child, not herself. She tries to address the child's problem, and in the process becomes over-protective and fuses with the child. Fusion with one child is usually greatest; however, other siblings may be involved to a lesser extent (Bowen, 1978; Shealy, 1988). Because the process is not focused evenly on all of the children, it is possible for some children to have less capacity for differentiation than their parents, others to have the same capacity, and others may attain higher differentiation. Bowen (1971) has contended that the family projection process is a universal phenomenon to some degree. He wrote that "it alleviates the anxiety of undifferentiation in the present generation at the expense of the next generation" (p. 398).

Emotional Cutoff

Emotional cutoff concerns "the way people separate themselves from the past in order to start their lives in the present generation" (Bowen, 1978, p. 382).

As an adult child starts an independent life, the manner in which separation from parents is handled is referred to as "emotional cutoff" (Bowen, 1978). The child may choose to handle separation by creating physical distance from the parents, or the separation may be handled by psychologically cutting off the parents (Shealy, 1988). According to Okun and Rappaport (1980), "How well people differentiate themselves from their original families, how much emotional attachment remains, is a critical determinant of how individuals handle all subsequent emotional relationships" (p. 119).

Multigenerational Transmission Process

Multigenerational transmission process concerns the "projection of varying degrees of immaturity (undifferentiation) to different children when the process is repeated over a number of generations" (Bowen, 1971, p. 398). The concept of multigenerational transmission process extends the family projection system to more than one generation. One child in a family (who is the focus of parental anxiety) grows up with low levels of differentiation and marries someone of similar differentiation, and the process is continued into another generation (Bowen, 1978). Several generations may pass before severe symptomatology is seen in a child.

Sibling Position

Sibling position concerns the influence that birth order has on personality characteristics (Bowen, 1978). Sibling position in a family provides information about personality profiles of individuals. The functional expectations for children in the various birth orders (oldest son, youngest child, etc.) are ingrained into the structure of the family down through the generations. These patterns transcend cultural values and can even be observed in the animal kingdom. Bowen (1971), writing about sibling position, observed that a person's order of birth may be used to understand the family emotional process of not only the present nuclear and extended family, but also that of the past generation.

Societal Regression

Societal regression concerns society's response to increasing societal anxiety. Efforts are directed toward allaying the anxiety of the moment, resulting in dysfunction (Bowen, 1978). Bowen contends that chronic societal anxiety and societal crises cause responses in society that are similar to those seen in families, but to a greater extent. As societal anxiety becomes more chronic, society reacts by making decisions to decrease the symptoms of the moment. This "band-aid approach" fails to alleviate the problem, and a cyclical phenomenon occurs.

Examples of Concepts Relevant to Clinical Practice

All of the concepts of Bowen's theory have some relevancy for clinical practice. An example of seven of these concepts will be presented. The focus of this chapter is on the nuclear family; therefore, societal regression will not be discussed.

Differentiation of Self

After the birth of Betty Jo, Barbara devoted all of her time and energy to her daughter. The two were seldom separated. At 18 years of age, Betty Jo married Barry, a 39-year-old man who lived next door. The couple lived in Barry's house, and Betty Jo spent each day with her mother. The marriage lasted 3 months, at which time Betty Jo moved back home with her parents. The difficulty in the marriage was related to Betty's inability to form a separate identity from her mother.

Triangles

Ralph was referred to the school counselor because of poor school performance. The initial interview with the parents revealed intense conflict between the two, which recently had accelerated. It was at this time that they began to focus on Ralph's school performance and to expect higher grades from him than they had done in the past. They had "triangled" in Ralph, in an effort to reduce the anxiety generated by the conflict in the marital relationship.

Nuclear Family Emotional System

Jim, who is very assertive, independent, and extroverted married Joan who is shy, dependent, and a loner. Jim made most of the decisions and Joan submissively complied. When stress occurred in the relationship, Jim became more assertive and spent more time with friends, while Joan became more withdrawn. Jim believed that Joan was rejecting him when she would not go to parties with him; Joan believed that her husband was not available to her when she was feeling so alone. As long as the relationship was unstressed, the patterns of interaction (dependent/independent) provided the couple with a balance in the relationship. However, when stress occurred, this balance was interrupted and the couple began to have marital conflict.

Family Projection Process

During Mary's pregnancy she experienced a great deal of anxiety and ambivalence about the pregnancy. When her daughter Pamela was born, the infant was fretful and difficult to care for. Mary spent more and more time caring for Pamela, and thus an intense relationship developed between the two. Pamela had difficulty in school, finding it hard to make friends. When she graduated from high school and went to college, she continued to have difficulty making friends and began to feel anxious and insecure. These feelings interfered with her school work and she was referred to the school counselor.

Emotional Cutoff

As a teenager Robert wanted to rebel against the guidelines set up by his parents. His friends experimented with drugs and he would have liked to join them. However, he believed his parents to be very powerful and feared their displeasure. He was unable to express his feelings to them and grew up feeling very resentful. He married at 19 years of age, moved to a distant city, and through the years that followed initiated very little contact with his family of origin. When his mother and father would come to visit their son and his wife, Robert would work long hours, thus avoiding his parents.

Multigenerational Transmission Process

Although there were four children in the Miller family, Nancy was considered to be her mother's favorite. She liked to help her mother and was not happy when she was playing with other children. As she grew older, she never dated or socialized with people her age. When Nancy was 30 years old, her mother died. A year later, Nancy married Tim, who also had a very close relationship with his mother. He had lived at home and taken care of his invalid mother until she died. He met Nancy at church and after they discovered how much they had in common with each other, they began dating.

After their daughter Barbara was born, Nancy and Tim repeated the pattern that had occurred in their childhood homes. They focused a lot of attention on their daughter and limited her interactions with other children. As Barbara grew up, she displayed little interest in the normal activities of her age group, preferring to go on outings with her parents. Thus, the multigenerational transmission process is evident in these two generations and may well show up in yet another generation if Barbara marries.

Sibling Position

John, 16-years-old, was the oldest son in the Nelson family. His parents placed a great deal of responsibility on him. They expected him to make good grades, work a full-time job, and watch his younger brothers when he was at home. Now that he had begun to drive, he was expected to chauffeur his younger brothers to all of their various activities. When John questioned these responsibilities, his father told him, "this is what the oldest son in a family always does." Recently John had begun to fight with his two younger brothers and last night he told his mother that he was going to leave home.

The family members' perception of behaviors that are appropriate for the first born (sibling position) appears to have influenced the functioning of this family.

Major Relational Statements

This section of the chapter will present major concepts in Bowen's theory and their relationship to each other. The concepts are interlocking and cyclical in nature. However, for ease of discussion, they are presented in a sequential order. Additionally, specific relationship statements will be presented to demonstrate how the theory can be tested.

A person's level of differentiation is developed in the environment of the nuclear family. When there is impairment in the nuclear family emotional system, it is likely that at least some members of the family will exhibit low levels of differentiation. The level of differentiation is also influenced by the birth order (sibling position) of an individual. The patterns of emotional functioning in a single generation (the nuclear family) are then passed on to future generations (multigenerational transmission process).

According to Bowen, two people of similar levels of differentiation meet and marry. At this point, the nuclear family is created. This two-person system may be stable as long as there are few stressors in the relationship. As the stressors increase in the couple's relationship, anxiety increases. When anxiety reaches a certain level, the two-person system triangles in the most readily available third person. Frequently, this third person is a child in the family.

As triangling occurs, the family projection process also occurs. One of the parents, generally the mother, projects anxiety to the triangled child, who in turn has increased anxiety levels in response to the mother's anxiety. The mother responds to the child, who she now considers impaired, and fuses with this child. The child becomes emotionally attached to the mother and thus develops a low level of differentiation. This situation results in an unresolved emotional attachment, which eventually leads to emotional cutoff. This emotional cutoff may be a physical cutoff, such as geographical distancing, or an emotional cutoff, such as limited interaction between family members who live in the same city. Many relational statements can be proposed that link Bowen's concepts together. Examples of testable relationship statements are:

1. The lower the level of differentiation of the husband and wife, the more intense will be the emotional fusion in the nuclear family.
2. The lower the level of differentiation of an individual, the more intense will be the degree of emotional cutoff and unresolved attachment to the family of origin.
3. The greater the degree of emotional cutoff of an individual from the family of origin, the more likely there will be emotional fusion in the person's nuclear family.
4. The greater the degree of stress experienced by a family, the more likely that triangling will occur.

IMPLICATIONS OF BOWEN'S THEORY FOR NURSING PRACTICE

This section of the discussion covers the use of Bowen's theory in nursing practice with families. Factors to be assessed, methods of assessing families, theory-specific diagnoses, the care plan, and evaluation of the care plan are presented.

Factors to be Assessed and Methods of Assessment

The overall goal of Bowen's theory "is to follow the total family through time with a focus on related events in interlocking fields" (Bowen, 1966, p. 366). Because Bowen's theory uses a systems approach to the study of families, theory-based assessment focuses on the family as a system. This means that assessment must include data about the family of origin of one or both spouses, if possible. One method of securing this data is through the development of a genogram. A genogram is a diagram or map of a family depicting the relationships between members and the significant events that have occurred in the lives of the members.

Other methods of assessment would include direct interviewing and observation of communication patterns of the family. These two techniques will provide information about the family's level of functioning. Assessment data will be obtained from the family about presenting problems of the nuclear family, functioning of the marital couple, and information about the extended family.

An example of an assessment guide will be presented with the theoretical basis for the specific information to be obtained from family members.

Assessment Data

I. Nuclear family
   A. Symptoms of presenting patient
      1. When symptoms first appeared
      2. What was going on at appearance of symptoms
      3. Onset of symptoms in relation to dates and events in parental/marital relationship

II. Functioning of the nuclear system since marriage
   A. Contact with extended family: (closeness/distance/emotional contact)
   B. Change in residence
   C. Purchase of home
   D. Occupation (successes/failures)
   E. Members in household
      1. Date of birth (in order)
      2. Place of birth

   F. Functioning of nuclear family members
      1. Physical
      2. Emotional
      3. Alcohol use
      4. Behavior/character disorder
      5. School problems

Theoretical Basis

". . . want to know about the functioning in the nuclear family field and then how the functioning of the extended family field intergears with the nuclear field. A good starting point is a chronological review of the symptom development . . . with specific dates and circumstances at the time of each symptom eruption" (Bowen, 1966, p. 364).

"The internal system also responds to the emotional fields of the extended families and to the reality stresses of life. The goal is to get a brief chronological review of the internal system as it has interresponded with outside forces" (Bowen, 1966, p. 365).

"Important ego mass changes accompany the birth of children" (Bowen, 1966, p. 365).

"Most families seek help when there is dysfunction in one or more of the three stress areas of the nuclear family system: (1) marital conflict, (2) dysfunction in a spouse, or (3) dysfunction in a child" (Bowen, 1966, p. 364).

G. Stress and anxiety (chronic or acute)
  1. Dates
  2. Sources
  3. Resources
  4. Coping strategies
  5. Feeling-fantasy system of family members

The way families handle anxiety determines if symptoms occur. Usual mechanisms for handling acute anxiety may not work when chronic anxiety is present (Okun & Rappaport, 1980).
"It is desirable to get readings on the feeling-fantasy system of various family members at stress points . . ." (Bowen, 1966, p. 365).

H. Serious illness or death in extended family

"Many symptomatic eruptions can be timed exactly with other events in the nuclear family fields" (Bowen, 1966, p. 364).

I. Mother's fantasy system before and after birth of child

"A check on the family projection process is often easy by asking about the mother's fantasy system before and after the birth of the child" (Bowen, 1966, p. 365).

J. Levels of differentiation
  1. Administer the Family System Personality Profile (Garfinkel, 1980)

". . . the level of differentiation and the degree of anxiety in the emotional field are the two primary variables for understanding symptom development and progression . . ." (Kerr, 1981, p. 254).

  2. Number of feeling statements ("I feel")

Intellectual functioning is so submerged that they cannot say "I think" or "I believe" (Bowen, 1978).

  4. Communication patterns
  5. How separated from family of origin

"One important aspect of differentiation of self is the process of dealing with unresolved emotional attachments with parents" (Jones, 1980, p. 54).

  6. Ability to make long-term goals

People with low levels of differentiation have difficulty making long-term goals (Bowen, 1978).

III. Extended family
   A. Parents/grandparents
      1. Occupation
      2. Marital relationship
      3. Health status
      4. Contact with members

"Exact dates, ages, and place are very important. The occupation of the grandfather and a note about the marital relationship and the health of each grandparent provide key clues to that family ego mass" (Bowen, 1966, p. 366).

"In general, a life style developed in the family of origin will operate in the nuclear family . . ." (Bowen, 1966, p. 366).

   B. Siblings of marital couple
      1. Names
      2. Birth order
      3. Dates of birth
      4. Occupations
      5. Places of residence

"Information about each sibling includes birth order, exact dates of birth, occupation, place of residence . . ." (Bowen, 1966, p. 366). Birth order can be influential on adult behavior (Bowen, 1978).

Theory-Specific Diagnoses

Nursing diagnoses which are specific to Bowen's theory address dysfunction in the family system. The response component of the nursing diagnosis can be observed in the marital couple, in either spouse, or in one or more of the children in the family. However, the etiology component of the nursing diagnosis is always associated with a disturbance in the entire family system.

Response Component

Couple—marital conflict, spouse abuse, inappropriate role performances, extramarital affair, disrupted communication patterns.
Spouse—depression, substance abuse, low self-esteem, inappropriate parenting skills, aggressive behavior.

Child—poor school performance, acting out behaviors, impaired relationships with peers, impaired relationships with siblings, psychosomatic complaints.

Etiology Component

Etiologies for family nursing diagnoses are derived from seven of Bowen's major concepts: differentiation of self, triangles, nuclear family emotional system, family projection process, emotional cutoff, multigenerational transmission process, sibling position.

Sample Nursing Diagnoses

Examples of theory-specific nursing diagnoses using the Bowen theory.
Couple

1. *Reluctance of husband and wife to make family decisions related to being the youngest child in their families of origin.*
   "In a marriage of two youngest children both are inclined to feel a little burdened by responsibility and having to make decisions. Neither is quick to take initiative and there can be a paralysis in the decision-making process" (Kerr, 1981, p. 251).
2. *Marital conflict of husband and wife related to fusion in the nuclear family emotional system.*
   "The fusion of the pseudo-selfs of the husband and wife into a common self may occur when two people of low levels of differentiation marry. The fusion results in anxiety for one or both of the spouses. The most universal mechanism for dealing with fusion is emotional distancing from each other" (Bowen, 1978, p. 377).

Spouse

1. *Difficulty in establishing satisfying relationships with others related to low levels of differentiation of self.*
   "People with low levels of differentiation of self pursue a lifelong quest for the 'ideal' relationship" (Okun & Rappaport, 1980, p. 116).

2. *Depression related to emotional distancing from family of origin.*
A person who has unresolved emotional attachment to the family of
origin may internalize the symptoms when under stress, and show
evidence of depression (Bowen, 1978).

Child

1. *Poor school performance of child related to triangled relationship
   with parents.*
   "When tension increases in a two-person system, the system will
   involve the most vulnerable other person to become a triangle"
   (Bowen, 1978, p. 373).
2. *Anxiety in the child related to the family projection process.*
   "The child may respond with anxiety to the mother's anxious behavior" (Okun & Rappaport, 1980, p. 118).

Care Plan

After the nursing diagnosis has been formulated, a plan of care will be
developed with goals and intervention strategies that are consistent with the
Bowen Theory. Client goals and predicted outcomes are formulated and
nursing interventions and specific nursing actions are planned. Interventions
focus on cognitive processes to help the family change their emotional
system.

Plans are made to see spouses together. This arrangement involves the
"two most important people in the family" (Bowen, 1971, p. 410). It allows
the nurse therapist to work on two important concepts—self-differentiation
and triangles. According to Bowen (1971) one of the goals of therapy is to
help individual members of the family to achieve higher levels of self-
differentiation. By seeing the spouses together this goal is easier to achieve.
Bowen (1971) writes that differentiation of self "involves the definition of
self in relation to other selfs about important life issues important to self. The
other spouse is one of the best people for the introduction of important
issues" (p. 410).

As tension increases between the couple, the therapist may become a
potential triangle in their relationship. If the nurse therapist will focus on
process rather than content of the therapeutic session, there will be less
chance that he or she will become triangled into the family's emotional

system. Another means of avoiding triangling is for the nurse to keep the tension low and to focus on the dynamics of the system rather than individual dynamics. If the couple can have contact with a third person who can relate to both without taking sides and becoming triangled into the relationship, the tension between them will resolve.

Bowen (1971) believes that the therapist must plan to spend some time in "defining the details of a system of minor-appearing stimuli that trigger intense emotional responses in the other spouse" (p. 412). Because most stimulus-response reactions are out of conscious awareness, the couple must be taught how to identify the most prominent stimulus-response mechanisms. This stimuli-response system must be defined in a step-by-step sequence to assist the couple to identify it and to change their behavior. The following is an example of a stimulus-response reaction.

A couple were discussing plans for the weekend. During the discussion the wife mentioned a visit to her parents. The husband's facial expression became closed and rigid. The wife continued to talk about plans but the husband remained rigid and withdrawn, not contributing to the discussion. In a discussion with a nurse therapist the following week, the wife complained about the husband's lack of interest in "anything but work." It was only after discussing the wife's reasons for believing this and examining the last time she had felt this way that the husband was able to identify what had triggered his withdrawal: the mention of a visit to his wife's parents, which he did not want to make but he was afraid of her displeasure if he stated this.

Interventions should be planned that will facilitate the couple's clear expression of thoughts. To do this the therapist will help one spouse to verbalize a clear thought, then ask the other spouse for a response to what was verbalized. Then the first spouse is asked to respond to the second spouse's thoughts. This question and answer process continues throughout the sessions, keeping questions calm and low-keyed. Each spouse is encouraged to talk directly to the therapist rather than to each other (Bowen, 1971). If either spouse begins to demonstrate emotions, the nurse therapist will try to get the other spouse to think about the emotion rather than express it. This approach to therapy helps the couple to express feelings openly and spontaneously and sets the stage for the beginning of differentiation of self.

Therapeutic interventions to be used, according to Jones (1980), involve clarifying the marital relationship and teaching the family about the emotional system. "The therapist communicates important principles of systems theory and makes indirect suggestions about directions the family may find profitable in resolving problems" (Bowen, 1971, p. 415). Teaching should come when tension between the couple is low and should be done in a manner that does not involve the nurse therapist in the family emotional system.

The nurse therapist demonstrates the taking of "I" positions, which helps the couple develop a greater degree of differentiation. This is done by the nurse therapist defining his or her own beliefs during interventions with the couple. Then the couple will begin to do the same in relation to each other (Bowen, 1971).

Although the presenting problem of an individual family member may not be dealt with directly, Bowen's theory assumes that changes in any part of the system will bring about change in the total system. Bowen (1971) states that there are many techniques of family psychotherapy but that most "involve shifting from individual dynamics to systems thinking and avoiding emotional fusion in the family emotional system" (p. 414).

The nurse who uses Bowen's theory should develop plans that address four main functions of the nurse therapist: defining and clarifying the relationship between spouses, keeping self de-triangled from the family emotional system, teaching the function of emotional systems, and taking "I" position stands (Okun & Rappaport, 1980).

Implementation of the Care Plan

The nurse documents the nursing actions that were carried out. This documentation should show the extent to which the care plan has been carried out and the type of behavior change that has occurred in the family. Behavior change in the family will be indicated by decrease in marital conflict.

Evaluation of the Care Plan

A comparison will be made between the predicted outcomes and the actual outcomes in order to determine product outcomes. Process outcome will be evaluated by examining the documentation of the extent to which the nursing actions were actually implemented and by determining change in the etiology component—that is, change in the ability of the family to separate from the family of origin.

THEORY-DIRECTED NURSING CARE
FOR THE ATKINS FAMILY

The discussion will now center on the use of Bowen's theory in working with the family described in the clinical case vignette. The steps of the nursing process model (Ziegler, Vaughan-Wrobel, & Erlen, 1986) are illustrated.

Assessing

Several concepts from Bowen's theory may be identified from the case data. Information provided in the case study gives a broad overview of the family as well as specific data about the family's functioning. The assessment guide that was presented in an earlier section of this chapter was used during the initial interview with the Atkins family. Only the data which are significant for the application of the concept of triangles would be used to develop the plan of care for this family.

Patrick's regressive behavior is evidence that the couple has triangled him into their two-person system. The couple is unable to deal with the tension within their relationship and another person (Patrick) is added to the system in an effort to reduce the tension. Richard and Alicia are focusing their attention and concerns on Patrick's regressive behaviors, thus taking the focus from the marital relationship.

Diagnosing

The following diagnosis was formulated based on the data presented in the case situation.

Patrick's Regressive Behavior Related to Triangling in the Family Relationship

Response: Patrick's regressive behavior

Subjective Data
"I want to sleep with you."

Objective Data
Patrick's thumb sucking.
Patrick's crying when parents argue.

Etiology: Triangling in the Family Relationship

Subjective Data

None presented

Objective Data

Alicia focuses on Patrick's behavior. Alicia changes subject when the nurse talks about the couple's relationship.
Alicia and Richard do not talk to each other.

Planning

Based on the subjective and objective data for the response and etiology component of the nursing diagnosis, goals and predicted outcomes have been formulated. Nursing interventions and specific nursing actions are presented.

Goal: Patrick will demonstrate fewer regressive behaviors.
Predicted Outcomes: After one month, Patrick will

1. Stop sucking his thumb
2. Request to sleep with parents will be made less than once a week
3. Instances of crying will decrease

Nursing Interventions:

1. Help the couple to clarify their marital relationship
2. Teach couple ways to interact with each other that will facilitate their relationship and decrease triangling behavior
3. Role model behaviors that will prevent the pair from incorporating the nurse into a triangle.

Nursing Actions

1. Only husband and wife will be seen by nurse.

2. Exploration of Alicia and Richard's relationship.

3. During sessions, encourage couple to talk to nurse, rather than each other.

Rationale

The marital relationship "is fundamental to the creation and resolution of family problems" (Squyres, 1987 p. 172).

The entire family system will change if the parental system changes (Bowen 1966).

By speaking to the therapist, the couple is able to clarify and define their relationship (Okun & Rappaport, 1980).

4. Discourage couple from talking to each other at home about their problems.

Bowen found that emotional disclosure often caused greater problems.

5. Have couple talk about emotion-laden subjects in a low-keyed calm manner.

A calm intellectual approach provides each spouse the opportunity to know the other in a way they might not otherwise have (Okun & Rappaport, 1980).

6. Ask direct questions from one spouse to the other about important issues between them rather than focusing on Patrick's behavior.

The purpose is to enable one of the couple to "express a clear piece of thinking, then to ask the spouse for a response" (Bowen 1971, p. 411).

7. Nurse refrains from becoming emotionally involved (triangled) in the relationship.

The nurse assumes a nonemotional stance to demonstrate that potentially strong emotional issues can be handled without deep emotional investment (Squyres, 1987, p. 172).

8. Teach couple about triangles and how the couple can handle their conflict.

"It is important to teach the family how to differentiate and clarify their values, and how to resolve family problems" (Okun & Rappaport, 1980, p. 124).

9. Coach the couple in ways to avoid triangling Patrick into their conflict.

10. Have couple take "I" position.

When an "I" position can be maintained even for a short period of time, there is a decrease in the intensity of the attachment between the other two, with more long-lasting decrease in the intensity of the triangle (Bowen, 1966, p. 373).

11. Use "reversal." Comment on the less obvious or opposite side of the an issue while picking up on the slightly humorous aspect. An example would be: When Alicia talks about Richard not caring, the nurse could respond, "I suppose Richard came to see you in the hospital because he likes the smell of them."

"A reversal or comment that focuses on the opposite side of the issue or that picks up the humorous side of the situation can decompress the mounting tension" (Bowen 1971, p. 413).

<table>
<tr>
<td>12. Have the couple talk about feelings, rather than expressing them.</td>
<td>Distinguishing between intellect and feelings and the verbalization of these in the presence of the other spouse provides for the rapid establishment of communication between spouses (Bowen, 1971).</td>
</tr>
</table>

Implementing

Documentation indicates the following client behaviors:

1. After one month of therapy Patrick continues to suck his thumb occasionally.
2. Patrick no longer requests to sleep with his parents.
3. Patrick cries less frequently.

Documentation indicates the following implementation of the nursing actions:

1. Because of a family emergency, the nurse met with the couple three times during the month, rather than four times as planned.
2. Only the husband and wife were seen in the sessions.
3. The nurse role-modeled nonemotional behavior when emotion-laden issues were discussed.
4. The nurse taught the family about emotional systems and how to clarify their values.
5. After three sessions, Alicia and Richard began talking more to the nurse during the sessions rather than to each other.
6. The couple reported that they rarely talked to each other at home about their problems, rather waiting until they were in the presence of the nurse.
7. Alicia and Richard were able to talk about some emotion-laden topics in a calm manner. However, they still continued to shout at each other when the topic of Richard's drinking came up.
8. The nurse asked direct questions about important issues concerning the use of alcohol, the death of the baby, and the move from New York. The couple responded to these direct questions.

9. Both on a few occasions during the sessions were able to take "I" positions.
10. The nurse used "reversal" in presenting the less obvious side of the issue that was being discussed. Alicia said that she was able to see that Richard had really wanted to see her when he came to the hospital, after the therapist remarked "I suppose Richard came to see you in the hospital because he likes the smell of hospitals."
11. Although the couple continued to argue, they began to talk about their feelings after the emotional display had dissipated.

Evaluating

Product Evaluation (Extent that Goals and Predicted Outcomes were Met)

1. After one month of therapy, Patrick continued to suck his thumb occasionally. This behavior suggests that the time frame for cessation of the thumb-sucking behavior may have been unrealistic.
2. Patrick no longer requests to sleep with his parents; therefore this outcome was achieved.
3. Patrick cries less frequently when his parents argue; this outcome was achieved.

Process Evaluation

Nurse Focus (extent that planned nursing interventions and nursing actions were implemented).

1. The nurse was unable to keep one appointment with the family. An unexpected personal crisis was the reason for the failure to keep the appointment. The family was notified; however, the nurse remains concerned that this missed appointment may have affected the final outcome of the sessions.
2. The nurse carried out the plan of meeting only with the husband and wife. Patrick was not included in the sessions.

3. The nurse was able to control her own emotions when discussing sensitive issues. Thus, she role-modeled appropriate behavior for the couple.
4. The nurse carried out the role of teacher in presenting Alicia and Richard information about emotional systems.

Client Focus (extent that etiology component of the nursing diagnosis statement was modified).

1. Alicia and Richard carried out the nurse's instructions to talk to her during the sessions, rather than to each other.
2. The couple reported that they had been able to carry through with the proposed action of not talking to each other at home about their problems, except on a few occasions.
3. The couple was able to focus more frequently on the conflict in their relationship. However, occasionally they returned to a discussion of Patrick's behaviors.
4. The couple was able to respond to the nurse's direct questions about important family issues. They did not try to change the subject or take the focus off the discussion of emotion-laden issues.
5. Each one was able to take "I" positions on several occasions. However, they still were having difficulty with self-individuation issues.
6. After the nurse used "reversal," Alicia was able to see Richard in a different light and realized that he really had wanted to see her when he came to the hospital after the baby was born.
7. The couple was more able to talk about their feelings; however, they continued to display strong emotions when interacting with each other. They will need to continue to work on expressing feelings without displaying their inner emotions.

SUMMARY

This chapter has dealt with a description and application of Bowen's family theory with a client family. Bowen's theory, which views the family as a system, allows the nurse to consider the complexity of the family unit when providing nursing care for families. Nursing care based on Bowen's family theory is quite different from the care that would be provided to individual members of a family who are exhibiting problems. The nurse makes the assumption that changes in any member of the family will affect other family members. Therefore, the nurse works with the family as a unit in the implementation of the nursing process.

REFERENCES

Bowen, M. (1966). The use of family theory in clinical practice. *Comprehensive Psychiatry, 7,* 345–374.

Bowen, M. (1971). Family therapy and family group therapy. In H. I. Kaplan & B. J. Sadock (Eds.) *Comprehensive group psychotherapy,* (pp. 394–421). Baltimore: Williams & Wilkins.

Bowen, M. (1978). *Family therapy in clinical practice.* New York: Jason Aronson.

Garfinkel, H. N. (1980). *Family systems personality profile: An assessment instrument based on the Bowen theory.* Unpublished doctoral dissertation, California School of Professional Psychology, Fresno.

Jones, S. L. (1980). *Family therapy: A comparison of approaches.* Bowie, MD: Brady.

Kerr, M. E. (1981). Family systems theory and therapy. In A. S. Gurman & D. P. Kniskern, *Handbook of family therapy* (pp. 226–264). New York: Brunner/Mazel.

Minuchin, S. (1974). *Families and family therapy.* Cambridge, MA: Harvard University Press.

Okun, B. F., & Rappaport, L. J. (1980). *Working with families: An introduction to family therapy.* North Scituate, MA: Duxbury Press.

Satir, V. (1967). *Conjoint family therapy.* Palo Alto, CA: Science and Behavior Books.

Satir, V., Stachowiak, J., & Taschman, H. (1983). *Helping families to change.* New York: Jason, Aronson.

Squyres, E. (1987). Approaches to the self: An examination of the work of Bowen and Jung. *Family Therapy, 14,* 165–178.

Ziegler, S. M., Vaughan-Wrobel, B. C., & Erlen, J. A. (1986). *Nursing process, nursing diagnosis, and nursing knowledge: Avenues to autonomy.* Norwalk, CT: Appleton-Century-Crofts.

SUGGESTED READINGS

Minuchin, S. (1965). Conflict-resolution family therapy. *American Journal Orthopsychiatry, 28,* 278–286.

Minuchin, S. (1967). *Families of the slums.* New York: Basic Books.

Minuchin, S. (1974). *Families and family therapy.* Cambridge, MA: Harvard University Press.

Minuchin, S., Rosman, B., & Baker, L. (1978). *Psychosomatic families.* Cambridge, MA: Harvard University Press.

Satir, V. (1965). The family as a treatment unit. *Confina Psychiatrica, 8,* 37–42.

Satir, V. (1972) *Peoplemaking.* Palo Alto, CA: Science and Behavior Books.

Chapter 6

Erikson's Theory of Psychosocial Development

Caryl E. Mobley and Judy Johnson-Russell

Promotion of optimal development in children has long been a concern of nurses. Enhancing children's physical and psychosocial growth through recognizing developmental needs and giving parents anticipatory guidance is a hallmark of holistic pediatric nursing practice.

The following case presentation involving 5-year-old Joanna and her family illustrates how nurses can assess children and their environments to promote optimal development. The three theories that will be considered for guiding use of the nursing process are Beavers' systems model of family functioning, Coopersmith's self-esteem theory, and Erikson's theory of psychosocial development. Erikson's theory will then be explored in-depth as it relates to this case.

CLIENT CASE

Joanna Cooke is a 5-year-old female who is brought into the well-child clinic by her mother to update her immunizations prior to starting school. Ms. Harris, the nurse examining her, finds that her height is in the 25th percentile and her weight is in the 10th percentile. Joanna lives with her mother and father, a 3-year-old brother named Jeff, and 6-month-old twin sisters. Both parents are in their mid-twenties and neither completed high school.

Joanna's father works at odd jobs, does not bring in a steady income, and is rarely home except to sleep. Her mother works part-time for a housecleaning service. When Mrs. Cooke is at work, the children are cared for by various neighbors. Mrs. Cooke says that Joanna has not had any health problems other than the usual colds and flu that children get. Ms. Harris does not find any problems on Joanna's physical examination. When she checks the 5-year-old items on the Denver Prescreening Developmental Questionnaire-Revised, Joanna is not able to perform many of the items. The nurse decides to make a home visit to further assess Joanna's development and the home environment.

The Cookes live in a poorly kept four-room, two-bedroom house. When Ms. Harris walks in, she notices a ball and a few old toy cars on the floor. The only printed material visible is a copy of a weekly tabloid. During the visit Ms. Harris accompanies Mrs. Cooke into the bedroom that all four children share; the furniture is old but sturdy, with a crib that the twins share and a double bed that Joanna and her brother share. Several infant toys and a bottle containing brown liquid are in the crib.

As Ms. Harris begins to talk to Mrs. Cooke about Joanna, Mrs. Cooke says that her daughter is very quiet and easy to have around. She states, "It's a good thing too, because with Jeff and the babies, I don't have any time left for her." When you ask what Joanna likes to do, her mother responds "Oh, sometimes she plays in the backyard with her brother or by herself, but mostly she likes to watch TV." There are no children Joanna's age with whom she plays in the neighborhood. Mrs. Cooke adds, "She's real good with the babies; she feeds them and changes their diapers and watches them sometimes when I have to go out for a little while."

Ms. Harris proceeds to do developmental screening with Joanna using the Denver II. In the personal-social area, Joanna has a failure on one task she should be able to complete. She is able to perform all of the tasks for her age in the gross motor area but has difficulty with three out of four tasks in the fine motor area. Joanna is very hesitant to talk to the nurse and, when she does speak, she uses a very quiet voice and three- or four-word simple sentences. Joanna shows failures on three age-appropriate Denver II language items. Ms. Harris concludes that Joanna shows delays in language and fine motor abilities. Her mother says that this performance is typical for her. When questioned further, Mrs. Cooke adds that Joanna rarely asks questions or tries new things without a lot of encouragement.

Since the home visit has been made shortly after Joanna started school,

Ms. Harris asks Mrs. Cooke how the first 2 weeks went. Mrs. Cooke replies that it did not go well. Joanna came home crying one day but would not tell her mother what happened. The teacher called at the end of the week and said that Joanna was not doing her work with the rest of the class and did not play with the other children. When they had circle time, Joanna went off to the corner and would not join the group. Mrs. Cooke says, "I don't understand it; Joanna's so good at home."

PATTERNING CUES FROM THE CLIENT CASE

In examining this case closely, a number of cues present the picture of a child and family in need of nursing intervention. Mrs. Cooke is aware of some needs of 5-year-olds, such as getting immunizations to prepare for entering school and providing a home environment that allows for basic physical growth and health. At the same time, she seems to be overwhelmed by the task of caring for Joanna's younger siblings without much support from her spouse.

Joanna shows an ability to perform in one area in which she has received stimulation and instruction, namely, taking care of babies. In most other areas of development, she seems to be progressing well behind other children of her age.

Using these cues to ascertain the primary problem with which she is faced, Ms. Harris recognizes that she needs to help this family change a pattern of not enhancing child development to one of encouraging optimal development in the children. Thus, she is confronted with helping Mrs. Cooke optimize her limited time and financial resources to provide a home environment which will encourage her children to develop more competently.

SELECTED RELEVANT THEORIES

A number of family, developmental, and psychological theories can be applied to assist nurses in meeting this family's needs. Three specific theoretical perspectives that can be used to help organize this data and plan appropriate interventions are that of the family, using a family systems model (Beavers, 1977), or that of the child, using self-esteem theory (Coopersmith, 1967), or psychosocial developmental theory (Erikson, 1963).

Beavers' Systems Model of Family Functioning

A family systems approach to Joanna's problems assumes that the primary focus in need of intervention is not the child herself, but overall family functioning. The family is viewed as a dynamic interactive system. What affects one member of the family reverberates throughout the system affecting all members of the family. In addition, family systems functioning is related to how a family interacts with other social systems outside the immediate family. Beavers (1977) believes that there is a relationship between overall systems competence and the child's level of functioning. The case of the Cooke family reveals not only decreased levels of functioning for the child, but also hints that problems exist within the family system in general and with its ability to relate to society.

The Beavers' Systems Model of Family Functioning provides a model that is useful both for determining family competence and style and for planning interventions. Using this model, the family can be understood as existing on a continuum from healthy to midrange to severely dysfunctional, and on a stylistic dimension continuum from centripetal to centrifugal. Centripetal refers to the situation in which the family's primary source of emotional gratification rests within the family and centrifugal refers to the family that seeks emotional gratification from outside the family. Beavers, Hampson, and Hulgus (1990) say, "competent families with young children are more centripetal, while with adolescents ready to leave home, they become more centrifugal" (p. 3). Understanding family functioning and style "provides a useful map for locating essential systems characteristics associated with family and individual psychological and behavioral functioning" (Beavers et al., 1990, p. 81).

Assessment using the Beavers' Systems Model of Family Functioning can be accomplished using the Beavers Interactional Scales. These include measures of family competence, family style, and a self-report family inventory. They can be completed in the home setting (Beavers, 1989) and they combine information from the nurse's observations with the family's perceptions of their own functioning.

A nursing diagnosis that would be pertinent to the Cooke's case using assessment of family functioning would be "altered growth and development related to a dysfunctional family system." Nursing interventions for the Cookes would be based on the findings from the assessment tools and could include increasing effective communication between the parents, strengthening the parental coalition, and recognizing and enhancing developmental needs of all family members.

Coopersmith's Self-Esteem Theory

Having a favorable attitude toward oneself is closely associated with personal satisfaction and effective functioning in our society (Coopersmith, 1967). Thus, the development of positive self-esteem in children is relevant to their total development as individuals.

Coopersmith (1967) defined self-esteem as "the evaluation which the individual makes and customarily maintains with regard to himself; it . . . indicates the extent to which the individual believes himself to be capable, significant, successful, and worthy" (pp. 4–5). This personal judgment of worthiness develops prior to middle childhood and remains relatively stable thereafter. It may vary across different areas of experience. For example, children have been found to develop a concept of self in several different areas, namely physical, cognitive, and social (Damon, 1983).

Based on a review of theorists and investigators who expounded on self-esteem, Coopersmith (1967) concluded that four factors contributed to its development: the amount of respect, caring, and acceptance one receives from those who are most significant; the successful experiences one has had, along with the recognition they bring; one's own interpretation of these successes based on individual values and aspirations; and the manner in which a person responds to negative appraisals of others and thus defends his or her self-esteem.

Using the data supplied by the present case study, one nursing diagnosis derived from self-esteem theory could be "poor self-esteem related to lack of respect and acceptance from parents." In relating this nursing diagnosis to Coopersmith's factors, the nurse can assert that, while Mrs. Cooke may be a very caring individual, demands on her time and energy have not allowed her to demonstrate much interest and attention to Joanna. On the other hand, based on the one successful experience about which data is given, care of the infants, Joanna has received recognition. The last two factors are difficult to evaluate in this case, particularly with a young child who is not very verbal and does not interact much with others. Nursing interventions that would be appropriate to this theoretical view of Joanna's case would include discussing with parents how they can show caring, respect, and acceptance to a 5-year-old and teaching them how to give Joanna experiences at which she can be successful.

Erikson's Theory of Psychosocial Development

The final theory to be discussed, and the one used to fully develop the case study, is the theory of psychosocial development put forth by Erik Erikson

(1963). Erikson has been grouped with the neo-Freudians and, as such, is concerned with the psychoanalytic approach to dealing with psychopathology. However, rather than focusing on libidinal influences on development as Freud did, Erikson views development within the context of the family and its historical-cultural heritage (Maier, 1965).

Development of the individual is influenced by three essential variables— irreversible inner biological processes, cultural influences which specify the rate of development and which biological processes are most important, and the individual's response to societal demands (Maier, 1965). This broad view of developmental influences, as well as the psychosocial focus of the theory, has made Erikson's theory very relevant to practitioners in the health sciences, including nurses. The theory lends direction to guide the nurse in identifying those aspects of child development in which to intervene.

DESCRIPTION OF ERIKSON'S THEORY OF PSYCHOSOCIAL DEVELOPMENT

Erikson introduced his stage theory in 1963 and has dealt with various aspects of it in other texts (1962, 1968, 1974). In addition, numerous other authors, including Maier (1965), have served as secondary sources in summarizing and discussing Erikson's stage theory. In this brief description of Erikson's theory, the authors examine underlying concepts that lay the foundation for utilizing this theoretical framework in clinical practice.

Major Concepts

The evolution of Erikson's developmental theory has involved three important concepts—sequential developmental stages, developmental conflicts or crises, and the formation of identity (Table 6.1).

Table 6.1.   Selected concepts of Erikson's Theory of Psychosocial Development

Sequential Developmental Stages
   Trust versus Mistrust
   Autonomy versus Shame and Doubt
   Initiative versus Guilt
Developmental Crises
Formation of Identity

Theoretical Definitions of Major Concepts

Sequential Development Stages

During development the individual moves through various periods, or stages, in which particular activities, or tasks, are accomplished. Erikson's theory explores the patterning of those particular tasks which are pertinent to psychosocial development throughout the lifespan.

Erikson's lifespan approach to development involves eight developmental stages. These are: trust versus mistrust, autonomy versus shame and doubt, initiative versus guilt, industry versus inferiority, identity versus role confusion, intimacy versus isolation, generativity versus stagnation, and ego integrity versus despair. Here the authors will only discuss the first three as they relate to this particular case study.

Trust versus mistrust. This first stage of development involves approximately the first year of life. The task of this stage is establishing an enduring sense of trust within the infant that basic needs will be met. The child who successfully establishes this trust is willing to allow the caregiver to be out of sight without undue anxiety. In addition, the infant will be able to grow psychologically and accept new experiences. Mutual regulation between the infant and caregiver evolves as the parent learns to read the infant's needs and the infant is able to read the parents' emotional and attitudinal behaviors. This trust must involve not only the caregiver, but also the environment. Parents need to establish an environment in which the child feels safe, loved, and cared for. By the end of the first year, then, the child should be able to view self as a separate entity within the environment where needs are met by those who share that environment.

If this trust is established, the foundation is set for the child to move onto the next stage. Conversely, infants who have not adequately developed a sense of trust are not prepared to fully accomplish the tasks of succeeding stages.

Autonomy versus shame and doubt. Because the child has developed trust and gained a strong attachment to the caregiver by the end of the first year of life, this sense of dependency creates in the child concern about one's capabilities and the need to assert oneself and be independent of the caregiver. This stage coincides with the child's newly found abilities to become mobile and explore the world. The culturally determined setting in which this stage takes place is within the give-and-take relationship between the child and parents. Within limits that are safe for the child, the toddler who gains a sense of autonomy is allowed some freedom and independence. The degree and type of freedom allowed the child varies from culture to culture. Children who do not gain this sense of control through appropriate experiences with autonomy develop a sense of shame about their inability and doubt that they are able to become independent people.

Initiative versus guilt. The sense of control over self gained during toddlerhood leads to an expectation by children that they are able to assume some responsibility for the environment and master new tasks that are within their abilities. They becomes very skilled at moving around in the environment and using language, which, in turn, increases the children's interactions with other people and with the social and cultural world. Preschoolers start to gain insight into their roles and opportunities in relation to society. When a sense of initiative does not develop appropriately, a sense of guilt about not becoming actively involved in the social world can impede children's further psychosocial development.

Developmental Crisis

The second concept that is evident throughout Erikson's work is that of developmental crises or conflicts. His developmental framework focuses on human anxiety and the areas of disturbance that cause anxiety. He studies "human growth from the point of view of the conflicts, inner and outer, which the vital personality weathers, re-emerging from each crisis with a sense of inner unity . . . and an increase in his capacity "to do well" according to his own standards and to the standards of those who are significant to him" (Erikson, 1968, p. 92).

In each of the developmental stages, Erikson identified a crisis related to a task which must be accomplished in order for the individual to move onto the next stage. From the standpoint of this concept, development was expressed in terms of gaining competency in a struggle between two opposite outcomes.

Formation of Identity

Striving for identity was a focus of much of Erikson's work. He viewed the formation of identity as a process which is at the core of the individual and the core of the culture (Erikson, 1968). The formation of identity involves judgment of self, formed in light of judgments made by others. Erikson saw identity as ever-changing, with increasing differentiation and more inclusiveness as the person becomes aware of judgments made by a increasingly greater variety of people.

Erikson felt that identity becomes the key psychosocial challenge during adolescence, but remains an important consideration in even the earliest stage of child development (Damon, 1983). While the beginning of identity formation is primarily unconscious during infancy, over time individuals become more aware of their identities (Erikson, 1968). In infancy, the child learns to recognize one's separateness from others. As trust evolves, the child learns to identify himself or herself as separate from the environment and people within the environment. An extremely relevant aspect of identity formation during toddlerhood is learning to control one's body and bodily functions (Damon, 1983). The child who gains a reasonable and appropriate degree of autonomy also gains a sense of identity as one who has control over one's body and bodily functions.

Preschoolers who take the initiative to explore roles and opportunities are forming a sense of purpose and a positive self-identity. Preschool children begin to imagine about their roles in the world, a world which is limited only by the boundaries of the child's own imagination. If the child takes the initiative to explore various possibilities, identity formation tends to encompass a positive view of social roles.

Examples of Concepts Relevant to Clinical Practice

One clinical setting in which these concepts can be clearly observed is the hospital playroom. Tommy is a 10-month-old who is playing with an infant toy with his mother. He remains on her lap, responds happily when his mother shows enjoyment of his ability to play with the toy, and watches other children playing (awareness of self as a separate individual). He is perfectly content (trust) until a nurse who has not cared for him approaches (crisis). He abruptly stops playing, turns in toward his mother (trust), and hides his head.

Near Tommy is Sarah, $2\frac{1}{2}$ years old, who is putting together a puzzle at the table. Her mother is sitting nearby talking with another mother. A few minutes ago, Sarah's mother saw she was having trouble with one piece and tried to help. Sarah pushed her mother's hand out of the way and said "No, I do it" (autonomy). You have noticed that every few minutes Sarah glanced at her mother to make sure she was still there (struggle between dependence and independence). As the nurse entered the room (crisis), Sarah left her puzzle and went to sit on her mother's lap; she watched the nurse intently until she saw that the nurse had come for another child. Then, Sarah resumed her position at the table playing with the puzzle (autonomy).

Betsy is a 4-year-old who has been playing with the child life specialist and two other children. They have a bear that they are "giving shots to" and examining. Betsy pretends that the bear is having the same surgery she has recently undergone and describes the entire experience to the child life specialist (initiative). A little while later, when her father enters the room, she runs over to greet him, takes him over to where she has been playing, and goes through the entire procedure with him (initiative), showing a great deal of pride (sense of self).

Major Relational Statements

These three concepts can be related to each other to demonstrate a coherent representation of psychosocial development. In each of the eight developmental stages there is a crisis which must be reconciled in order for the individual to move onto the next stage. The developmental crisis represents the focal point of each stage. The formation of identity serves as the potential goal for each stage. Both the sequence and rate at which individuals achieve the stages impacts development. If a developmental crisis is not dealt with at the right time and in the right sequence, not only will that particular aspect of development be hindered, but the progression through subsequent developmental stages will also be endangered. However, with reasonable socialization and appropriate guidance from the environment, development will progress.

The challenge for the individual, then, is to resolve crises in a manner that will allow development to progress in its orderly fashion. If the crisis is resolved in a positive manner, the stage is set for progression to the next developmental step and a more mature level of identity. If the crisis is not resolved in an appropriate manner, negative aspects of the personality will become apparent and the individual's identity formation will be hindered.

IMPLICATIONS OF ERIKSON'S PSYCHOSOCIAL DEVELOPMENTAL THEORY FOR CLINICAL PRACTICE

Erikson's theory can be used in all phases of the nursing process to develop effective plans of care for children. Since development is viewed from an environmental as well as a biological perspective, intervention with whole families becomes an important factor.

Factors to be Assessed and Methods of Assessing

Aspects of development which should be assessed are derived from all three concepts reviewed. The sequential developmental stages are the organizing force behind the developmental assessment. In order to understand a child's current developmental level, nurses must comprehend past developmental patterns. Therefore, they should question parents and older children about patterns of parent-child interaction, responsiveness to social stimuli, emotional sensitivity, and social maturity. Since physical and motor development can impact socioemotional development, a history of the child's growth in these areas is also important. Out of this assessment should come a sense of the child's developmental history.

The second aspect of development which should be assessed involves the child's handling of crises or conflicts. Nurses can question parents about how their child managed problems they were expected to encounter at the previous stage. For example, if a toddler is being assessed, parents would be questioned about how their child reacted to separation from parents. Parental discipline strategies, and the child's reaction to them, would be appropriate areas of inquiry for parents of preschoolers. Nurses should also ask parents about situations that are currently anxiety-provoking for their child and what the child does to cope with these situations. Parents and older children may be asked a general question about the child's competency in handling day-to-day problems.

Finally, the child's level of identity formation is assessed. This evaluation focuses on those aspects of identity which are expected to evolve during a particular developmental period. An example would be the preschool period, when children are gaining identity in terms of sex roles and their role in society. Assessment in this area can involve observations of the child's behavior and comments about his or her own identity, as well as questioning parents about their observations of the roles the child takes in the family and the child's perceptions of these roles.

The resulting assessment should reflect a holistic approach to the situation and include the child, family, and all relevant aspects of the environmental situation. The child needs to be considered from the developmental perspective—what is appropriate for the child at a particular age and ability level, especially in terms of self-identity, what tasks should the child already have mastered, and what developmental challenges can the child be expected to encounter next. The family also needs to be considered from a number of viewpoints: configuration and roles; financial and social resources; intellectual, educational, and cultural background; and communication patterns. Finally, the environment of the child needs to be examined. This includes physical resources of the home and other people and institutions of which the child is part, such as school, church, and peer group activities.

While no assessment tools specific to Erikson's theory of psychosocial development have been found, several instruments will give indications of development that would be applicable. Tests such as the Denver Developmental Screening Test, Denver II, Vineland Social Maturity Scale, and, for older children, the Self-Esteem Inventory can be very helpful in assessing areas related to psychosocial development.

Theory-Specific Diagnoses

Erikson's theory of psychosocial development can be used in generating a variety of nursing diagnoses that can be individualized to the particular child's developmental level and problem area.

Response Component

Since the individual is the focus of psychosocial development theory, the response component of the nursing diagnosis will concentrate on the child. The following list suggests possible responses commensurate with Erikson's theory, but is certainly not an exhaustive list.

1. Inadequate achievement of age-specific developmental task (specify)
2. Disturbance in self-esteem
3. Impaired social adjustment
4. Personal identity disturbance
5. Altered role performance
6. Inappropriate behavior
7. Ineffective coping behavior

8. Anxiety
9. Fear
10. Hopelessness

Etiology Component

Since environmental factors play an important role in psychosocial development, the etiology component of the nursing diagnosis may involve the child, family, or both. Thus, this etiology can focus on a great variety of factors that influence the development of children. Some of these are:

1. Mental, emotional, or physical limitations of the child
2. Inadequate resolution of previous developmental conflicts/crises
3. Parental lack of knowledge about development, parenting, or needs of children
4. Ineffective parent-child interaction
5. Inappropriate parental discipline
6. Parental abuse or neglect
7. Inadequate or inappropriate environmental stimulation
8. Lack of financial, social, emotional, or spiritual resources
9. Parental mental, emotional, or physical limitations
10. Inefficient parental time management

Sample Nursing Diagnoses

A few of the infinite number of possible nursing diagnoses follow:

1. *Lack of trust (autonomy, initiative, etc.) related to ineffective parent-child interaction.*
   "The general sense of trust, furthermore, implies . . . that one has learned to rely on the sameness and continuity of the outer providers . . ." (Erikson, 1963, p. 248).
2. *Anxiety related to lack of identity-building experiences.*
   "There are, therefore, few frustrations in either this [trust vs. mistrust] or the following stages which the growing child cannot endure if the frustration leads to the ever-renewed experience of greater sameness and stronger continuity of development, toward a final

integration of the individual life cycle with some meaningful wider belongingness" (Erikson, 1963, p. 249).

3. *Impaired social adjustment related to lack of adequate social support systems.*
   Since development of the individual takes place in a social arena and is strongly influenced by the demands of society (Erikson, 1963), lack of appropriate social support can thwart development.

4. *Disturbance in self-esteem related to parental lack of knowledge about needs of children.*
   "The style of one's individuality . . . coincides with the sameness and continuity of one's meaning for significant others in the immediate community" (Erikson, 1968, p. 50).

5. *Inappropriate child behavior (specify) related to inadequate parenting skills/discipline.*
   "It is important to realize that in the sequence of his most personal experiences, the healthy child, given a reasonable amount of proper guidance, can be trusted to obey inner laws of development" (Erikson, 1968, p. 93).

6. *Hopelessness related to a parent-child relationship that does not encourage establishment of trust (or of autonomy or initiative, etc.).*
   Erikson sees hope "as being the first and the most basic" virtue which emerges "from the interplay of individual growth and social structure" (1968, p. 233).

Care Plan

When using Erikson's theory, nursing interventions would focus on enhancing the psychosocial development of the child. Any factors in the environment that can have an impact on the development of the child need to be taken into consideration. This may include physical and psychological aspects of the home and other entities such as schools and community organizations of which the child is a part. Thus, an overall objective for nursing care would be to change the child's environment in such a way as to help the child gain and/or maintain a sense of adaptation and identity (Erikson, 1968).

Nurses can be involved in this process by helping the child and/or family set appropriate goals and look toward the outcomes they expect to occur. Erikson's theory can be used to guide this process, using its specification of the attributes of one who has achieved successful mastery of each of the developmental crises. Therefore, goals can be set to guide the attainment of these attributes.

By the end of the first stage of development, the attribute that Erikson feels is essential for development is the sense of trust between the infant and the primary caregiver. Therefore, a goal for this stage would be the development of a trusting relationship between parent and child. Specific predicted outcomes would be related to observable behaviors that denote a trusting relationship, including the infant's responsiveness to parental cues and the parent's consistency in meeting the needs of the infant. A goal relevant to the second stage of development, autonomy versus shame and doubt, would be that the child gain the interest and self-reliance to explore an environment that is appropriately stimulating to a young child. Predicted outcomes for parents might include providing age-appropriate toys for the child and a safe environment in which to play. The child would demonstrate autonomy by freely exploring the toys and returning to the parent briefly for reassurance of proximity and affection. Similar goals and predicted outcomes could be developed for the remaining developmental stages.

Interventions are then devised that focus on achieving the goal by influencing factors that lead to the problem the nurse identified. These interventions can involve the entire environmental milieu of the child to shore up the child's inner sense of identity and outer response to the environment. In helping the family optimize development of children, the nurse must be cognizant of characteristics and capabilities of the child, family members, and any others who have an impact on the child. Interventions may include teaching, encouraging parent-child interaction, helping parents select appropriate materials and stimulation, reassuring parents about their ability to parent, and seeking appropriate community support for families.

Delineation of nursing actions involves the use of appropriate resources to achieve the goals set forward. Erikson's theory does not specify actions which, when taken, will help restore the individual to a sense of equilibrium and positive identity. Rather, knowledge about how children develop, how children and families should function, and psychosocial processes can be used to develop actions that move the child and family toward meeting the goals.

Implementation of the Care Plan

The nurse's role in implementing the plan of care is that of collaborator with the child, family, and any others who are involved in optimizing the development of the child. In many cases the nurse can act as an organizer and manager to see that all aspects of the plan are being performed in an orderly manner. However, the nurse's primary role is that of an advocate for the child, to be someone that the child knows has his or her best interest in mind, and someone who will strive to assist the child in reaching an optimal level of development.

Evaluation of the Care Plan

Monitoring of the child's ongoing developmental progress is important when evaluating movement toward the goal. This evaluation can involve a number of processes related to determining how close the child's actual outcomes are to the predicted outcomes (product outcome evaluation) and how effective the nursing interventions are in modifying the etiology component of the nursing diagnosis (process evaluation). As with earlier parts of the nursing process, all people involved in helping the child reach the goals should be involved in the evaluation process. The methods for evaluating the product and process may include informal observations of and interviews with the child and family, or more formal standardized testing of the child.

THEORY-DIRECTED NURSING CARE FOR THE COOKE CASE

The nursing process, utilizing Erikson's theory of psychosocial development, can be applied to the case study involving Joanna Cooke. Much of the data outlined in this illustration points to a number of problem areas for this child.

Assessing

In terms of assessment data for Joanna, while her physical growth and health status appear to be within normal limits, she has delays in language and fine motor development. She has had very little experience with other children outside her family, is "very quiet," and rarely asks questions. She spends her days watching TV and playing by herself. Joanna shows little initiative in trying new things. However, she has shown ability to help take care of her baby sisters. Adaptation to school has proven to be difficult for her; Joanna is not doing her work or interacting with the other children, and she came home from school crying one day.

Joanna's family also has many needs. Both parents are young (early twenties) and neither has a high school education. Mr. Cooke is rarely present and does not seem to be involved in the family. Mrs. Cooke is responsible for raising four children, maintaining the home, and working part-time. When Mrs. Cooke is working, there is no consistent caregiver for the children.

The home environment in which Joanna is being raised is inadequate for the developmental needs of children. There are few age-appropriate toys and no printed material for children is present. Joanna shares a room with her three younger siblings.

Diagnosing

Although a number of nursing diagnoses could be written that would be consistent with these data, the following was selected to illustrate the use of the nursing process with this case.

Delay in Development of Initiative Related to Inadequate Levels of Environmental Stimulation

The following specific subjective and objective data validate this nursing diagnosis.

Response: Delay in development of initiative

Subjective Data	Objective Data
Joanna is "very quiet."	Joanna has difficulty with age-appropriate fine motor and language tasks on the Denver II.
Joanna's performance on the Denver II is "typical for her."	
Joanna "rarely asks questions."	Joanna is very hesitant to talk.
Joanna "rarely tries new things without a lot of encouragement."	

Joanna "came home from school one day crying" and would not tell her mother what happened.
Joanna "was not doing her work in class."
Joanna "went off to the corner and would not join the rest of the group."

Etiology: Inadequate levels of environmental stimulation

Subjective Data

"With Jeff and the babies, I don't have any time left for her."
"She mostly likes to watch TV."

Objective Data

Cookes live in a poorly kept small house.
A ball and a few old toys are visible. The only printed material visible is a weekly tabloid. There are no children Joanna's age with whom she plays in the neighborhood.

It is obvious from this data that further testing of Joanna to determine specific deficit areas is necessary. However, since the lack of environmental stimulation is quite evident, Ms. Harris can begin to plan her intervention without waiting for more definitive results.

Planning

Based on these data, Ms. Harris starts to plan her nursing care by setting a response-focused overall goal (delay in development of initiative).
Goal: Joanna will take the initiative to interact with other children and seek stimulation appropriate to her developmental level. Specific, time-referenced predicted outcomes related to this goal follow.

Predicted Outcomes:

1. Within 2 weeks, Joanna will take part in circle time in her classroom.
2. Within one month, Joanna will interact every day with at least one child at home or on the playground.
3. Within 3 months, Joanna will ask questions and initiate activities without encouragement from others.

Using the etiology component of the nursing diagnosis (inadequate levels of environmental stimulation), nursing interventions and nursing actions are formulated to increase the environmental stimulation Joanna receives.

Nursing Interventions:

The nurse will identify ways in which Joanna's family can make their home environment more stimulating at an appropriate developmental level for Joanna and her siblings.

The nurse will work with Joanna's teacher and other appropriate people in the school setting to design and set up a program that encourages Joanna's participation in classroom activities and with peers.

Nursing Actions	**Rationale**
1. Teach Mrs. C. about child development appropriate for her children's age groups.	Appropriate guidance of a child entails "the proper rate and the proper sequence" of interaction with the environment (Erikson, 1968, p. 93).
2. Help Mrs. C identify resources for obtaining toys and written materials for her children.	Toys and written material are part of a child's "complex 'milieu' which permits a human baby not only to survive but also to develop his' potentialities for growth and uniqueness" (Erikson, 1968, p. 222).
3. Demonstrate ways Mrs. C. can make educational toys from objects found around the house.	Preschool children "will find pleasurable accomplishment in wielding tools and weapons, in manipulating meaningful toys" (Erikson, 1963, p. 256).
4. Help Mrs. C. organize her time to accomplish household tasks and have time to play with her children.	"In connection with comprehensible games and work activities a companionship may develop between . . . mother and daughter, an experience of essential quality in worth" (Erikson, 1968, p. 121).
5. Assist Mrs. C. in identifying activities she can do to increase her children's curiosity and initiative.	The child "must emerge with a sense of initiative as a basis for a realistic sense of ambition and purpose" (Erikson, 1968, p. 115).

6. Meet with Joanna's teacher to determine appropriate people at school to work with Joanna.

In discussing good teachers, Erikson states, "For nothing less is at stake than the development and maintenance in children of a positive identification with those who know things and know how to do them" (1968, p. 125).

7. Arrange a planning session with identified people to select methods of helping Joanna begin to interact and take initiative.

"School seems to be a culture all by itself, with its own goals and limits, its achievements and disappointment." (Erikson, 1963, 259).

8. Select small behavioral goals and positive methods of discipline to encourage classroom participation.

In discussing the preschool period, Erikson says, "The child is at no time more ready to learn quickly and avidly" (1963, p. 258).

9. Determine, with the teacher's and mother's help, children who live nearby who may be potential friends for Joanna.

Regarding the stage into which Joanna is moving, industry is described as involving "doing things beside and with others" (Erikson, 1968, p. 126).

10. Arrange a simple activity to help Joanna and another child to get to know each other better.

Preschool children are "eager and able to make things cooperatively, to combine with other children for the purpose of constructing and planning" (Erikson, 1963, p. 258).

Implementing

The nurse, Ms. Harris, worked with Joanna, her mother, school teachers and personnel to help Joanna progress in her psychosocial development. Initially, she set up a time to meet with Mrs. Cooke at home when the twins were asleep and the other two children were not at home so there would be no distractions. Ms. Harris discussed the outcome of the initial testing of Joanna and the concerns that arose from the testing. She then assessed how much knowledge Mrs. Cooke had about child development, cleared up any inaccuracies, and answered questions. She supplied Joanna's mother with an easy-to-understand pamphlet highlighting early development and asked her to read it prior to their next visit. One week later, Mrs. Cooke and Ms. Harris met to discuss the pamphlet and visited an agency that supplies toys and books to needy children. The nurse talked about how to select age-appropriate toys and helped Mrs. Cooke select toys and picture books for her children. On her next visit to the Cooke home, Ms. Harris assisted Joanna's mother in going through objects in the home and identifying ways of combining and using objects to stimulate the children. She also showed Mrs. Cooke ways of reading to the children that would stimulate their curiosity and their interaction with the reader.

The purpose of Ms. Harris' next visit with Mrs. Cooke was to help her to organize her time to have more time with the children. Together they set up a schedule to try during the next week that included her work schedule, shopping, house cleaning, and routine child care activities. Time was set aside after the babies went to bed for Mrs. Cooke to do quiet activities and talk with Joanna and Jeff. Mr. Cooke came home during this meeting and Ms. Harris was able to discuss with him her findings and concerns about Joanna and ways she was working with Mrs. Cooke to help the family. He said he would help his wife more with the household chores and with taking care of the children.

During this period of time, Ms. Harris also met with Joanna's teacher, Mrs. Thomas. Mrs. Thomas shared some observations and concerns about Joanna and Ms. Harris showed the results of the screening tests done (Mrs. Cooke had given permission for this). Mrs. Thomas agreed to set up further educational, psychological, and developmental testing through the school system. Together they identified others in the school who would be appropriate to work with Joanna. These included the school counselor, the school nurse, the speech therapist, and the special education teacher.

On her next visit to the school, Ms. Harris met with this team and discussed her plan of care for Joanna; she then received their input into this plan. Together they set up short- and long-term goals for Joanna and discussed methods each could use to meet these goals. One short-term goal related to classroom participation was selected and broken down into specific behaviors that would be reinforced; methods of reinforcement were then decided upon.

At a group meeting the next week, progress toward this goal and the effectiveness of the reinforcement were discussed. Further goals pertaining to classroom behavior and interaction with peers and teachers were discussed, agreed upon, and broken into specific observable behaviors.

Ms. Harris met with Joanna's mother and teacher to share the goals and the plan that school personnel were implementing. Mrs.Cooke inquired about ways she could strengthen what was happening at school through interventions in the home; Mrs. Thomas and Ms. Harris both gave her some suggestions. The three of them then discussed children who lived in the area and who might be potential friends for Joanna. Two girls who lived within a few blocks were identified. Mrs. Cooke suggested that she and Joanna plan a picnic in a nearby park the next weekend and Joanna select which of the girls she would like to invite to come with them. Joanna could be involved in preparations and could find out what the other child liked to eat. Since Mrs. Cooke could take all of her children along, this would be a treat for everyone.

Evaluating

Product Evaluation (Extent that Goals and Predicted Outcomes were Met)

1. By the end of the sixth week, Joanna was beginning to ask a few questions about the stories her mother had read to her and had made her first trip to the library.
2. In school, the first short-term goal, having Joanna participate in circle, was accomplished by the end of the second week. While the success of other goals varied, Joanna started taking part in classroom activities consistently by the end of the first month, although she still spoke very little.
3. The picnic in the park was successful and Joanna and her friend started walking to school together and playing on the playground frequently.
4. By the end of 3 months, Joanna was reevaluated using the Denver II. She was able to pass all of the personal-social and gross motor tasks. She failed only one of the fine motor tasks. In the language area, she failed two of the age-appropriate items.

Process Evaluation

Nurse Focus (extent that planned nursing interventions and nursing actions were implemented).

1. Ms. Harris taught Mrs. Cooke about growth and development and appropriate ways of stimulating development in her children.

2. Ms. Harris organized and participated in planning school-based activities to encourage Joanna's development.
3. Ms. Harris helped Mrs. Cooke organize and evaluate a time management program for household tasks.
4. Ms. Harris assisted Mrs. Cooke in planning and organizing an activity for Joanna that reinforced her interaction with another child.

Client Focus (extent that etiology component of the nursing diagnosis statement was modified).

1. Ms. Harris found that Mrs. Cooke did have some knowledge about child development and was able to augment this knowledge. Mrs. Cooke showed interest in learning more through the thorough reading of the pamphlet and her questions.
2. Mrs. Cooke was able to select age-appropriate toys for each of her children after the initial visit and at a second visit. By the fourth visit, she had also made two toys for the babies out of objects found around the house.
3. On the third visit to the Cooke home, Mrs. Cooke reported that she had read to Joanna and Jeff three times the previous week. By the end of the sixth week, Mrs. Cooke was reading to the children almost every night.
4. At the end of the first month, Mrs. Cooke reported that her plan for getting her housework accomplished was working, that she felt less frustrated with getting everything done, and that she was able to spend about 15 minutes each with Jeff and Joanna on most evenings. She also was pleased that Mr. Cooke had stayed with the children several times while she did the shopping.
5. By the end of 6 weeks, Mrs. Cooke was able to provide age-appropriate stimulation for her children and had started to get Mr. Cooke more involved with the children.

SUMMARY

In this chapter the nursing process has been applied to a client case involving a young child and her family, using Erikson's theory of psychosocial development. Through the use of sequential developmental stages, developmental crises, and self-identity as the three principle concepts put forth by

Erikson, the theory was woven into each of the steps of the nursing process to show how a family can be assisted in assessing needs, setting goals, planning and implementing specific actions, and evaluating the effectiveness of the plan of care. Further, the role of the nurse in acting as an advocate for the child and in organizing key members of the child's social environment to advance psychosocial development were discussed.

REFERENCES

Beavers, W. R. (1977). *Psychotherapy and growth: Family systems perspective.* New York: Brunner/Mazel.
Beavers, W. R. (1989). Beavers systems model. In C. N. Ramsey (Ed.) *Family systems in medicine.* New York: Guilford Press.
Beavers, W. R., Hampson, R. B., & Hulgus, Y. F. (1990). *Beavers systems model manual.* Dallas: Southwest Family Institute.
Coopersmith, S. (1967). *The antecedents of self esteem.* San Francisco: W. H. Freeman.
Damon, W. (1983). *Social and personality development: Infancy through adolescence.* New York: W. W. Norton.
Erikson, E. H. (1962). *Young man Luther: A study in psychoanalysis and history.* New York: W. W. Norton.
Erikson, E. H. (1963). *Childhood and society* (2nd ed.). New York: W. W. Norton.
Erikson, E. H. (1968). *Identity: Youth and crisis.* New York: W. W. Norton.
Erikson, E. H. (1974). *Dimensions of a new identity.* New York: W. W. Norton.
Maier, H. W. (1965). *Three theories of child development.* New York: Harper & Row.

SUGGESTED READINGS

Lewis, J. M., Beavers, W. R., Gossett, J. T., & Phillips, V. A. (1976). *No single thread: Psychological health in family systems.* New York: Brunner/Mazel.
Miller, S. A. (1987). Promoting self-esteem in the hospitalized adolescent. *Issues in Comprehensive Pediatric Nursing, 10,* 187–194.
Reasoner, R. W. (1983). Enhancement of self-esteem in children and adolescents. *Family and Community Health, 6*(2), 51–64.
Stanwyck, D. J. (1983). Self-esteem through the life span. *Family and Community Health, 6,* 11–28.
Stuart, G. W., & Sundeen, S. J. (1991). Chapter 13: Alterations in self-concept. In *Principles and practice of psychiatric nursing* (4th ed.) (pp. 371–412). (4th ed.). St. Louis: Mosby Year Book.
Werner-Beland, J. A. (1986). Beavers' family systems approach: Reformulation for nursing. In A. L. Whall, *Family therapy theory for nursing: Four approaches* (pp. 127–141). Norwalk CN: Appleton-Century-Crofts.

Chapter 7

Lazarus' Theory of Coping

Kathleen M. Baldwin

$\mathbf{A}$ major nursing intervention is the enhancement of client coping skills during times of stress. The case of John Reynolds and his wife, Mary, will demonstrate how nurses may use Lazarus' (1976) Theory of Coping to help clients cope with a sudden change in health status and the long-term consequences of that change.

Following the case presentation, a summary of theories applicable to this case, Lazarus' (1976) Theory of Coping, Kobasa's (1979) Theory of Hardiness, and Mishel's (1988) Theory of Uncertainty, will be presented. By applying theoretical content from Lazarus' (1976) Theory of Coping with data from the case presentation, a plan for theory-directed nursing care is devised.

CLIENT CASE

John and Mary Reynolds have been married for 40 years and have three sons who are married and live in the same community. John, age 63, is an attorney. Mary, age 61, has never worked outside the home, but is very involved in community service, having served as chairperson for many projects. The couple is extremely active in their local church: John is a deacon; Mary is a Sunday School teacher. They have saved for retirement, are financially secure, and have been eagerly anticipating John's planned retirement at age 65. The only major crisis in their marriage occurred 6 years ago when John was involved in an auto accident and sustained severe injuries. He spent 3 weeks in intensive care, underwent two major surgeries, and had multiple blood transfusions. After a year of rehabilitation, he fully recovered.

Neither John nor Mary has had a physical exam in 2 years, but they consider themselves to be in good health for their respective ages. They are avid golfers and walk 2 miles a day for exercise. They are conscious of their diet, do not smoke, and drink alcohol in moderation.

The Reynolds' sons are married and live close by with their families. Two of the sons are attorneys and one is a university professor. John and Mary maintain a close, loving family relationship with all of their children and grandchildren. They frequently visit with each other, and John and Mary often keep their grandchildren in the evenings and over weekends.

Last week a colleague and close friend of John's required emergency surgery and used several units of blood. John immediately volunteered to donate a replacement unit for his friend and went directly to the blood donor center. He was subsequently notified by the blood donor center that his blood could not be used because it tested positive for the Human Immunodeficiency Virus (HIV). After consulting with their family doctor, John and Mary were referred to Dr. Brown, the physician who heads the community clinic which specializes in treating patients with Acquired Immune Deficiency Syndrome (AIDS).

Dr. Brown examined John and ordered laboratory tests, which subsequently confirmed the diagnosis of HIV infection. John became indignant and stated, "I know that there was some kind of error because I have never used intravenous drugs and I have never engaged in any type of homosexual behavior." Dr. Brown told John he had most probably contacted the infection from the blood transfusions he received after his accident. John and Mary became extremely upset and anxious when Dr. Brown suggested that Mary also needed to be tested. John demanded to know what the course of the illness would be, when he would recover, or when he would die. He became angry when Dr. Brown stated that those questions could not be answered because of the unpredictable nature of the disease. He shouted, "What kind of a doctor are you that you can't answer these simple questions. Find me someone who can!" Mary, who had been silent, began to cry uncontrollably, after stating that they would be ostracized by their family and friends.

Because of their response to the diagnosis, Dr. Brown strongly urged the Reynolds to meet with Nancy Miller, the director of nurses at the clinic, for counseling. Ms. Miller has been involved in the care of patients with HIV and AIDS for 5 years. She began working at the clinic shortly after her older brother, a hemophiliac, died of AIDS. She has been assigned the task of assisting John and Mary Reynolds to understand and cope with the fact that John contracted the HIV infection from a blood transfusion.

PATTERNING CUES FROM CLIENT CASE

After meeting with and interviewing the Reynolds, Ms. Miller begins to devise a plan for theory-directed nursing practice. Her first step is to identify cues from the interview that indicate problematic behaviors which would hinder satisfactory coping, as well as those behaviors available to John and Mary Reynolds that will assist them in adjusting.

Ms. Miller realizes that HIV seroconversion is a stress-producing event and that severe emotional responses to the diagnosis, although common, may hinder the development of problem-solving skills necessary for satisfactory coping. Problematic behaviors exhibited by the Reynolds include John's anger and Mary's tears. Fear of the social stigma attached to the diagnosis and fear of Mary's health status compound the Reynolds' emotional response to John's diagnosis.

Ms. Miller also identifies factors which should assist the Reynolds in coping with the diagnosis. Those factors include the Reynolds' lifestyle, involvement in church, history of successful marriage and child-rearing, close relationships with family and friends, and financial security.

SELECTED RELEVANT THEORIES

There are many theories that could be used to assist the Reynolds in coping. Three different theories, Kobasa's (1979) Theory of Hardiness, Mishel's (1988) Theory of Uncertainty in Illness, and Lazarus' (1976) Theory of Coping, will be discussed in order to demonstrate how different theories could be applied to the Reynolds' case. Each theory will result in different nursing diagnoses and different nursing interventions to assist the Reynolds.

Kobasa's Theory of Hardiness

Kobasa (1979) believed that people who handled high degrees of stress without succumbing to illness possessed a different personality structure than those who became ill. The name given to this personality structure was hardiness. According to Kobasa (1979), "hardy persons are considered to possess three general characteristics: the belief that they can control or influence the events of their experience; an ability to feel deeply involved in or committed to the activities of their lives; and the anticipation of change as an exciting challenge to further development" (p. 3).

A nursing diagnosis for the Reynolds' case using this theory would be "stress associated with HIV seroconversion related to ineffective use of hardiness characteristics." Nursing interventions to strengthen hardiness characteristics in Mr. Reynolds would include those that would increase his sense of control over the situation, would enhance his sense of commitment to the activities of his life such as his work, his church, and his family, and those that would encourage Mr. Reynolds to view his seroconversion as a challenge instead of a threat.

Mishel's Theory of Uncertainty in Illness

Mishel (1990) stated that uncertainty in illness "is the inability to determine the meaning of illness-related events and occurs in situations where the decision maker is unable to assign definite values to objects and events and/or is unable to accurately predict outcomes because sufficient cues are lacking" (p. 256). She described two appraisal processes, inference and illusion, which determine the value placed on uncertainty. Inference was defined as comparing the uncertainty to examples of similar situations. Illusion was defined as building a belief system with a positive outlook.

Based on results of the appraisal, the uncertainty is either viewed as a danger or an opportunity. When the uncertainty is viewed as a danger, coping strategies include mobilizing, which is comprised of direct actions, vigilance, and information seeking and affect-management which includes methods of faith, disengagement, and cognitive support (Mishel, 1988). When uncertainty is viewed as an opportunity, coping involves buffering strategies which serve to support the uncertainty and to block input of additional information that would change the uncertainty. Buffering strategies include avoidance, selective ignoring, reordering priorities, and neutralizing (Mishel, 1988). Successful use of the coping strategies associated with uncertainty viewed as either danger or opportunity results in adaptation.

A nursing diagnosis for the Reynolds' case using this theory would be "stress associated with HIV seroconversion related to viewing uncertainty as danger." Nursing interventions for Mr. Reynolds, based on this theory, would focus on the enhancement of mobilizing strategies to decrease the uncertainty. Methods for enhancement of mobilizing strategies for Mr. Reynolds might include asking him to become actively involved in planning and implementing his care (direct action), suggesting that he become attuned to small changes in his health status (increased vigilance), and/or encouraging him to increase his knowledge of HIV seroconversion and AIDS (information seeking).

If these were unsuccessful, then affect control strategies would be recommended to help Mr. Reynolds adapt to the emotional stress generated by the appraisal of danger. Methods for enhancement of affect control strategies might include suggesting that Mr. Reynolds continue to be actively involved in his church (faith), allowing him to withdraw (disengagement), and/or encouraging him to reevaluate his situation focusing on positive elements (cognitive support).

Lazarus' Coping Theory

Research contains evidence of two major views regarding the process of coping with stress. One view describes coping based on mastery of psychophysiological responses to stressors and is termed the traditional approach. The other view comes from psychoanalytical ego psychology and places importance on the cognitive processes used in coping with stressors.

Lazarus' Theory of Coping represents an example of a coping theory from psychoanalytical ego psychology. Within this framework two processes are viewed as critical when dealing with stress—the process of cognitive appraisal and the process of coping. Lazarus first presented the theory in 1966 and since then has been involved with colleagues in rigorous testing and refinement of the concepts. In addition to having a vast amount of research supporting the theory, the importance placed on cognitive appraisal makes this framework particularly attractive in the Reynolds' case.

DESCRIPTION OF LAZARUS' THEORY OF COPING

The reader is reminded that the description of Lazarus' theory is brief because of space restrictions. It is assumed that a reader who wishes to use

Lazarus' theory will seek out additional sources (especially primary sources) that describe the theory. Major primary sources of the theory include publications by Lazarus in 1976, Lazarus and Folkman in 1984, and Folkman, Lazarus, Dunkel-Schetter, DeLongis, and Gruen in 1986. Secondary sources, in which Lazarus' theory is presented in the context of nursing, include Pollock (1989), Nyamathi (1989), and Kirschling and McBride (1989).

Lazarus' theory is complex and addresses multiple concepts. The author, therefore, has selected those concepts that are believed to be most pertinent to the case presentation. These selected concepts are named, theoretically defined, clinical examples of the selected concepts are identified, and major relational statements are presented. Table 7.1 illustrates the major concepts of the theory.

Major Concepts

Lazarus' Theory of Coping contains three major concepts: stress, cognitive appraisal, and coping.

Table 7.1 Selected Concepts of Lazarus' Coping Theory

Stress
Cognitive Appraisal
   Types of Cognitive Appraisal
     Primary Appraisal
       Irrelevant Stressor
       Benign-Positive Stressor
       Stress-producing Stressor
         Threatening
         Challenging
     Secondary Appraisal
     Reappraisal
       Reapprasial That Is Not Defensive
       Defensive Reappraisal
   Factors Which Affect Cognitive Appraisal
     Personal Factors
     Situational Factors
Coping
   Forms of Coping
     Problem-focused Coping
     Emotion-focused Coping
   Factors Which Affect Coping
     Coping Resources
     Constraints Against Using Coping Resources

Theoretical Definitions of Major Concepts

Stress

Lazarus and Folkman (1984) defined stress as "a particular relationship between the person and the environment that is appraised by the person as taxing or exceeding his or her resources and endangering his or her well-being" (p. 18). They believed that stress resulted from an interaction of individual personal characteristics with the environmental event. The event which resulted in a stress response within the person was termed the stressor.

Cognitive Appraisal

Cognitive appraisal is defined as "a process through which the person evaluates whether a particular encounter with the environment is relevant to his or her well-being, and if so, in what ways" (Folkman et al., 1986, p. 992). The process involves evaluating the significance of all aspects of a stressor to determine the level of threat to one's well-being. Cognitive appraisal can be further classified into the types of cognitive appraisal and the factors which affect cognitive appraisal. The types of cognitive appraisal are primary appraisal, secondary appraisal, and reappraisal (Lazarus & Folkman, 1984).

Primary appraisal involves the evaluation of the nature of the threat. There are three outcomes of primary appraisal: the stressor is identified as irrelevant, the stressor is identified as benign-positive, or the stressor is identified as stress-producing. A stressor is deemed irrelevant when, after encountering it, the person determines that there is no threat to well-being. A stressor is deemed benign-positive when, after encountering it, the person determines that the outcome will, or is likely to, preserve or enhance well-being. A stressor is deemed stress-producing when, after encountering it, the person determines that there is a threat to well-being, that harm/loss will occur, or that a challenge exists.

Lazarus and Folkman (1984) stated that the difference between threat and harm/loss involves the concept of anticipatory coping. With threat, anticipatory coping (coping which precedes the event) may occur. In harm/loss there is no time for anticipatory coping. They differentiated between threat and challenge by explaining that not only is there a potential for growth or gain with a challenge, but that it is associated with pleasurable emotions. Threats are not accompanied by pleasurable emotions and are not viewed as having any potential for growth or gain.

Secondary appraisal involves the evaluation of the various coping options available. It is defined as "a complex evaluative process that takes into account which coping options are available, the likelihood that a given coping option will accomplish what it is supposed to, and the likelihood that one can apply a particular strategy or set of strategies effectively" (Lazarus & Folkman, 1984, p. 35). Lazarus and Folkman (1984) caution that these names are not meant to suggest that one process occurs prior to the second process, or that one is more important than the other. *Reappraisal* involves changing an appraisal based on new information received about the stressor. Reappraisal is divided into two types—not defensive and defensive. Reappraisal that is not defensive is viewed as virtually synonymous with appraisal, differing only in that it occurs after a previous appraisal. Defensive reappraisal is a self-generated process that attempts to reinterpret past events more positively. Lazarus and Folkman (1984) identified personal and situational factors which influenced the coping process. Personal factors influencing appraisal are the person's commitments and beliefs. Situational factors influencing appraisal include novelty, predictability, event uncertainty, temporal factors (imminence, duration, and temporal uncertainty), and ambiguity.

Coping

Coping is defined as a process of "constantly changing cognitive and behavioral efforts to manage specific external and/or internal demands that are appraised as taxing or exceeding the resources of the person" (Lazarus & Folkman, 1984, p. 141). Lazarus and Folkman (1984) identified forms of coping and factors which affect coping.

There are two forms of coping—problem-focused coping and emotion-focused coping. They believed that both forms of coping not only influenced one another during the coping process, but could impede or facilitate each other. With problem-focused coping attempts are made to alter or manage the stressor. With emotion-focused coping attempts are made to regulate the emotional response to the stressor.

Lazarus and Folkman (1984) identified two factors which affect the coping process—resources that assist with the coping process and constraints which impede it. Coping resources include health and energy, positive beliefs, problem-solving skills, social skills, social support, and material resources. Constraints against using coping resources include personal constraints, environmental constraints, and level of threat.

Examples of Concepts Relevant to Clinical Practice

Clinical examples of the selected concepts are presented.

A 19-year-old female college student is admitted to the hospital with symptoms of hyperglycemia. She is told that she is diabetic and that she will have to follow a strict diet, have morning and evening injections of insulin, and monitor her blood glucose levels several times a day in order to control her disease.

Primary appraisal of this situation results in the determination that it is stress-producing, because there is a threat to her well-being. Secondary appraisal of the situation results in anger and denial by the patient. After attending several diabetic classes and gaining a better understanding of diabetes mellitus, she reappraises the situation. She realizes that she can control her disease process and can lead a normal life once the diabetes is controlled. Reappraisal results in the determination that the situation is stress-producing, because a challenge exists—the challenge to gain control of her diabetes.

Coping options used after the reappraisal include problem-solving coping in order to gain control over the disease, and the use of emotion-focused coping to decrease emotional distress. Coping resources that could assist the client in adjusting to diabetes include her age and previously healthy physical state, her belief that controlling her diabetes is a challenge, her ability to use problem-solving skills, her ability to communicate well with others, the support of her family and friends, and her socioeconomic status. Constraints against using coping resources could include her preestablished beliefs about diabetes and chronic illnesses, the pressure of going to college and adjusting to a chronic illness, and the level of threat that the diagnoses of diabetes has to her well-being.

Major Relational Statements

The relational statements which serve to link the major concepts are presented.

1. It is not the nature of the stressor, but the person's cognitive appraisal of the stressor, which determines the degree of response.
2. An event that one person may appraise as stress-producing, other individuals may appraise as nonstress-producing.
3. Accurate cognitive appraisal results from the interplay of primary appraisal, secondary appraisal, and reappraisal, as well as identification and management of personal and situational factors which affect appraisal.
4. The degree of reaction produced by a stressor is related to the subjective appraisal each individual makes of the event.
5. The process of coping is process oriented, contextual, and serves to manage stress.
6. The two major functions of coping are to regulate stress-producing emotions and to alter the cause of stress.
7. The outcome of coping may be viewed as successful or unsuccessful based on the subjective judgment of the individual.
8. An effective coping process results from the appropriate use of problem-focused coping and emotion-focused coping as well as identification and management of resources which assist in the coping process and constraints which impede the coping process.

IMPLICATIONS OF LAZARUS' THEORY OF COPING FOR CLINICAL PRACTICE

In this section use of Lazarus' theory in nursing practice will be presented. Factors to be assessed, methods of assessing, theory-specific diagnoses, care planning, and evaluation of care are presented.

Factors to be Assessed and Methods of Assessing

The major concepts of the theory make up the factors to be assessed. First, an understanding of the client's cognitive appraisal of the stress-producing situation must be assessed. Assessment will include determining whether the client views the situation as irrelevant, benign, or stress-producing. If the client views the situation as stress-producing, the next step in the assessment process is to collect data to determine whether the situation is stress-producing because there is a threat to well-being, because harm or loss will occur, or because a challenge exists. The assessment process should then center on determining what the client views as coping options to the stress-producing situation and how successful the client feels these coping options will be. Following these steps, an assessment of personal and situational factors which influenced the appraisal process would be conducted.

Once the initial assessment of the appraisal processes used by the client is completed, it should be used as an initial data base from which ongoing assessments can be conducted. Ongoing assessments would focus on determining the individual's reappraisals of the situation as new information becomes available and/or the stress-producing situation alters. Differentiation between reappraisals that are not defensive and defensive reappraisals would be assessed and documented during the ongoing assessment process.

An initial assessment of the process of coping used by the client must also be conducted. Use of problem-focused methods of coping and emotion-focused methods of coping should be assessed and documented. The client's resources that will assist the process of coping, as well as the constraints which would impede coping, should be assessed and documented. As in the initial assessment for appraisal, this initial assessment will serve as a data base upon which ongoing assessments will be conducted. Changes in the stress-producing situation, the client's use of coping methods, resources, and/or restraints will be assessed in ongoing assessments.

There are several commercially available coping scales that could be used to assist in determining individual coping methods. One scale generated by nurses and based on Lazarus' theory is the Jalowiec Coping Scale (Jalowiec & Powers, 1981). This tool has been used in a variety of patient situations and has an established degree of validity and reliability.

Theory-Specific Diagnosis

Sample nursing diagnoses are presented that are specific to Lazarus' theory of coping. The processes of cognitive appraisal and coping are the focus for determining the etiology components of the nursing diagnoses.

Response Component

The major response component that can be identified by using Lazarus' theory is stress. Behavioral manifestations of stress could be used to generate a more specific response component and include anxiety, denial, anger, hostility, crying, depression, and hopelessness.

Etiology Component

Etiology components for the nursing diagnoses statements could reflect problems with appraisal of the stressful situation or problems with coping responses to the stress-producing situation. Examples of etiologies that may arise during appraisal of the stress-producing situation are:

1. The results of the primary appraisal are inaccurate.
2. There is a perceived threat to well-being.
3. The client erroneously believes that harm to or loss of well-being will occur.
4. There is ineffective identification of coping options (secondary appraisal).
5. There is an inaccurate reappraisal of the situation.
6. The client fails to accurately identify situational factors which influence the appraisal process.
7. The client fails to accurately identify personal factors which influence the appraisal process.

Examples of etiologies that might arise during the process of coping are:

1. The use of problem-focused coping methods is ineffective.
2. The use of emotion-focused coping methods is ineffective.
3. The use of problem-focused coping methods is impeded by emotional-focused coping methods.
4. The use of emotion-focused coping methods is impeded by problem-focused coping methods.
5. There is inaccurate identification and use of coping resources.
6. Constraints against using coping resources are perceived as insurmountable.

Sample Nursing Diagnoses

Examples of response and etiology components from Lazarus' Theory of Coping were used to form the following examples of nursing diagnoses.

1. *Stress (exhibited by anxiety) related to inaccurate primary appraisal.*
   "In any encounter with the environment, the key problem for the person is to make a series of realistic judgments about its implications for his or her well-being. . . . The mismatch between appraisal and what is actually happening can take two basic forms: either the person will appraise harm, threat, or challenge in instances and ways in which they do not apply; or the appraisal will reflect the failure to recognize harm, threat, or challenge in instances where they should be recognized" (Lazarus & Folkman, 1984, p. 186).
2. *Stress (exhibited by depression) related to impedance of problem-focused coping methods by emotional-focused coping methods.*
   ". . . two coping functions that are of overriding importance in nearly every type of stressful encounter: the regulation of stress (emotion-focused coping) and the management of the problem that is causing the stress (problem-focused coping). Coping effectiveness in a specific encounter is based on both functions. A person who manages a problem effectively, but at great emotional cost cannot be said to be coping effectively" (Lazarus & Folkman, 1984, p. 188).
3. *Stress (exhibited by hopelessness) related to ineffective use of problem-focused coping methods.*
   ". . . a negative belief about one's capacity to have any control in a situation, or about the efficacy of a particular stratagem to which one is committed, can discourage essential problem-focused coping efforts" (Lazarus & Folkman, 1984, p. 160).
4. *Stress (exhibited by anxiety) related to inaccurate reappraisal of the situation.*
   "Another factor that often makes the preparation for alternative outcomes difficult, if not impossible, is the mental confusion that can result from having to consider first one possible outcome and then another. When one cannot decide on a path of action and closure is unavailable, fear, excessive worrying and rumination, and eventually anxiety can result. The heightened anxiety (threat) is itself likely to interfere with cognitive functioning, making it even more difficult to cope" (Lazarus & Folkman, 1984, p. 92).
5. *Stress (exhibited by anger) related to the presence of constraints against using coping resources.*
   "Level of threat, in turn, influences the extent to which available resources can be used for coping. . . . The greater the threat, the more primitive, desperate, or regressive emotion-focused forms of coping tend to be and the more limited the range of problem-focused forms of coping" (Lazarus & Folkman, 1984, pp. 167–168).

6. *Stress (exhibited by denial) related to ineffective use of emotion-focused coping options.*

"Although emotion-focused processes may change the meaning of a stressful transaction without distorting reality, we must still consider the issue of self-deception, which is always a potential feature of this type of coping process. We use emotion-focused coping to maintain hope and optimism, to deny both fact and implication, to refuse to acknowledge at worst, to act as if what happened did not matter, and so on. These processes lend themselves to an interpretation of self-deception or reality distortion" (Lazarus & Folkman, 1984, p. 150).

7. *Stress (exhibited by hopelessness) related to an inaccurate identification and use of coping resources.*

"Viewing oneself positively can also be regarded as a very important psychological resource of coping. We include in this category those general and specific beliefs that serve as a basis for hope and that sustain coping efforts in the face of most adverse conditions" (Lazarus & Folkman, 1984, p. 159).

8. *Stress (exhibited by hostility) related to an inaccurate identification of coping options (secondary appraisal).*

"Secondary appraisals of coping options and primary appraisals of what is at stake interact with each other in shaping the degree of stress and the strength and quality (or content) of the emotional reaction" (Lazarus & Folkman, 1984, p. 35).

Care Plan

The major goal of a care plan based on Lazarus' Theory of Coping is that the client effectively manages the stress created by a stressor. In order to accomplish this, the client must form an accurate cognitive appraisal of the stressor and use effective coping methods.

Formation of an Accurate Appraisal

Interventions which would assist a client to form an accurate cognitive appraisal would be:

- Decrease ambiguity to decrease level of threat.
- Decrease vulnerability by decreasing personal and situational factors which affect appraisal.

- Change appraisals of threat into appraisals of challenge.
- Discuss all coping options available.

Lazarus and Folkman (1984) believed that ambiguity occurred when the information needed for an accurate appraisal was unclear or insufficient. "Whenever there is ambiguity, personal factors shape the understanding of the situation, thereby making the interpretation of the situation more a function of the person than of objective stimulus constraints" (Lazarus & Folkman, 1984, p. 104). Thus, for a client to develop an accurate appraisal of any stressful situation, clarification of areas of ambiguity must occur.

Psychological vulnerability also has the potential to adversely affect accurate appraisal. Lazarus and Folkman (1984) viewed vulnerability as a potential threat which becomes an actual threat when something a person values is jeopardized by a particular event. Thus, for a client to develop an accurate appraisal of any stress-producing situation, areas of psychological vulnerability must be minimized or balanced so they do not evolve into actual threats.

According to Lazarus and Folkman (1984) an appraisal of challenge, as opposed to an appraisal of threat, is accompanied by pleasurable emotions and focuses on the potential for individual growth while dealing with a stressor. Thus, the ability to change an appraisal of threat into an appraisal of challenge would result in a more positive client response to the stressor.

Discussion of all options of coping available to a client would allow for a more accurate appraisal of the client's ability to handle the stressor. By selecting coping options with the strongest chance for success, a client may be better able to view the stressor as a challenge instead of a threat.

Use of Effective Coping Methods

The following are interventions which would assist a client to use appropriate coping methods.

1. Enhance coping resources. Exploring each of these resources with a client and deciding which ones would most enhance coping with stress will increase coping effectiveness with any stressor.
2. Discuss constraints to coping and then eliminate or modify them. Exploring each of the constraints with a client and deciding which ones most hinder coping with stress will increase coping effectiveness with any stressor.

3. Consult with client to decide which forms of emotion-focused coping would be most beneficial.
4. Consult with client to decide which forms of problem-focused coping would be most beneficial.
5. Consult with client regarding the client's other agendas and determine which forms of emotion-focused and problem-focused coping would complement the client's other agendas.

Implementation of the Care Plan

Implementation of the care plan involves frequent counseling sessions during which the nurse and the client discuss measures to assist the client in coping with stress. Weekly, biweekly, or daily counseling should be arranged with the client, so that all aspects of the processes of appraisal and coping may be explored. Because Lazarus and Folkman (1984) viewed the processes of appraisal and coping as dynamic and constantly evolving, the implementation of interventions using this theory must be subject to frequent evaluations. Frequent evaluations permit adjustments in implementation of interventions, so they could address the dynamic, constantly evolving processes of appraisal and coping.

Evaluation of the Care Plan

The ultimate function of the coping process is the reduction or elimination of stress within the client, thus the effectiveness of the care plan must be evaluated by its ability to reduce or eliminate stress (product—outcome evaluation). According to Lazarus and Folkman (1984) there are three basic outcomes in successful coping with stress. The client who is coping successfully with stress will be able to function effectively at work and in social settings, have a high level of morale or life satisfaction, and be healthy somatically and not suffer from those physical conditions related to high levels of stress. Evaluation of the product of successful coping would mean identifying these attributes in a client who is coping with stress.

Because both cognitive appraisal and coping are viewed as constantly changing and evolving processes, the evaluation of the care plan must also be dynamic and must involve frequent assessments and adjustments whenever the client reappraises the stressful situation (process—client focused evaluation). Additionally, it is important to evaluate whether or not the nurse accurately identified stressors and effectively intervened to enhance the coping responses in the client (process—nurse focused evaluation).

THEORY-DIRECTED NURSING CARE
IN THE REYNOLDS' CASE

Lazarus' (1976) Theory of Coping is applied to the Reynolds' family. Each of the five steps of the nursing process are illustrated.

Assessing

The assessment data are organized under the categories of cognitive appraisal and coping. The following assessment data are relevant to the process of cognitive appraisal. In his primary appraisal Mr. Reynolds has correctly appraised his change in health status as stress-producing. He views the change as a threat to his well-being, thus anticipatory coping may result. Changing his appraisal from one of threat to one of challenge would allow for potential growth and decrease negative emotions. After secondary appraisal, Mr. Reynolds reacts with anger, Mrs. Reynolds reacts with fear. Personal factors which might have influenced Mr. Reynolds' appraisal include his personal beliefs about HIV and AIDS, his personal commitment to a health-promoting lifestyle, and his personal commitment to a church. Situational factors which might have influenced Mr. Reynolds' appraisal of the situation include novelty, since he never anticipated facing this type of problem, the uncertainty of the course of the disease, and the ambiguity or lack of clarity in the prognosis.

The following assessment data are relevant to the process of coping. Mr. Reynolds initially exhibited problem-solving skills by consulting his physician and a specialist after being informed of his HIV infection, demonstrating problem-focused coping. Mr. Reynolds reacted with indignation, anger, and denial, forms of emotion-focused coping, when the diagnosis was confirmed.

Mr. Reynolds has several resources to assist him in coping. The following are cues from the client case which indicate coping resources.

1. Health and energy evidenced by the fact that both John and Mary considered themselves to be in good health, the finding that John is asymptomatic at the present time, and the daily exercise and diet regime followed by the Reynolds.
2. Positive beliefs evidenced by the Reynolds' strong commitment to and involvement in their church.
3. Problem-solving skills evidenced by 40 years of successful marriage and the rearing of three sons.
4. Social skills evidenced by community involvement, religious involvement, and educational level.
5. Social supports evidenced by close relationships with their children, their activities in their church, and the programs of the local AIDS clinic that provide emotional support to individuals with HIV infection and their family members.
6. Material resources evidenced by the Reynolds' financial security.

However, Mr. Reynolds will also face constraints which will impede coping. Cues from the client case which indicate constraints against using coping resources include the following:

1. Personal constraints evidenced by the Reynolds' beliefs and fears about AIDS.
2. Environmental constraints evidenced by society's reactions toward individuals with AIDS and toward the largest groups at risk for infection (male homosexuals and intravenous drug abusers).
3. A high perceived level of threat evidenced by the Reynolds' reactions to the diagnosis and feelings about the consequences of having such a diagnosis.

Diagnosing

The following diagnosis was formulated based on the data presented in the clinical case.

Stress Associated with HIV Seroconversion Related to Inadequate Problem-Focused Coping Processes

Subjective and objective data to support the diagnosis are presented.

Response: Stress associated with HIV seroconversion

Subjective Data	Objective Data
"What kind of a doctor are you that you can't answer these simple questions? Find me someone who can!"	Exhibits indignation. Exhibits anger. Exhibits denial.

Etiology: Inadequate problem-focused coping processes

Subjective Data	Objective Data
"There must be some kind of error, because I have never used intravenous drugs or engaged in any type of homosexual behavior."	Demands to know disease course and outcome. Becomes angry when told the disease is unpredictable.

Planning

Based on the response component of the nursing diagnosis, "stress associated with HIV seroconversion," goals and predicted outcomes have been formulated.

Goal: Mr. Reynolds will feel less stress regarding HIV seroconversion.

Predicted Outcome: Mr. Reynolds will be able to discuss his HIV seroconversion without indignation, anger, or denial after 4 weeks of counseling.

Based on the etiology component of the nursing diagnosis statement, "inadequate problem-focused coping processes," the nursing interventions and nursing actions are planned.

Nursing Interventions
Modify Mr. Reynolds' primary appraisal through directed reappraisal, so that he views maintaining his asymptomatic state as a challenge instead of a threat and recognizes personal and situational factors which could assist or deter him.

Modify Mr. Reynolds' secondary appraisal through directed reappraisal, so that he identifies and uses effective problem-focused coping methods and recognizes resources that will assist him with coping and constraints that will impede him from coping.

Nursing Actions

1. Explain HIV seroconversion and AIDS and answer any questions Mr. Reynolds has concerning the disease in order to decrease ambiguity.

Rationale

"Ambiguity is present in one form or another in practically every type of human encounter. . . . In many instances ambiguity can be threatening, and the individual will seek to reduce it by searching for more information" (Lazarus & Folkman, 1984, p. 107).

2. Encourage Mr. Reynolds to express his concerns about his diagnosis.

"A threat appraisal can arise without the person clearly knowing the values and goals that are being evaluated as endangered, the internal or environmental factors that contribute to the sense of danger, or even that threat has been appraised" (Lazarus & Folkman, 1984, p. 52).

3. Assist Mr. Reynolds to identify parts of his disease process that he can control.

"Challenge appraisals are more likely to occur when the person has a sense of control over the troubled person-environment relationship" (Lazarus & Folkman, 1984, p. 36).

4. Discuss personal and situational factors which may affect Mr. Reynolds' appraisal.

"Many if not all person and situation factors have the potential to both contribute to and diminish threat. . . . It is extremely important to keep this characteristic in mind in any examination of person and situation antecedents of appraisal" (Lazarus & Folkman, 1984, pp. 114–115).

5. Assist Mr. Reynolds to identify all realistic judgments about the impact of HIV seroconversion.

"In any encounter with the environment, the key problem for the person is to make a series of realistic judgements about its implications for his or her well-being" (Lazarus & Folkman, 1984, pp. 185–186).

6. Allow Mr. Reynolds to express his anger and fear about his situation, then assist him to refocus his energy toward the manageable aspects of his illness.

7. Assist Mr. Reynolds to identify resources available to assist him to cope.

"Theoretically, problem- and emotion-focused coping can both facilitate and impede each other in the coping process" (Lazarus & Folkman, 1984, p. 153).

"We believe that information about resources can contribute to an understanding of why some people seem to be challenged more often than threatened, and fare better than others over the course of numerous stress-producing encounters" (Lazarus & Folkman, 1984, p. 170).

8. Assist Mr. Reynolds to identify and modify constraints against coping.

"The ways people actually cope also depend heavily on the resources that are available to them and the constraints that inhibit use of these resources in the context of the specific encounter" (Lazarus & Folkman, 1984, p. 158).

Implementing

Ms. Miller implemented the care plan for Mr. Reynolds during biweekly counseling meetings. Mrs. Reynolds also attended the meetings.

During the first week of counseling the Reynolds and Ms. Miller discussed Mr. Reynolds' diagnosis of HIV seroconversion. Ms. Miller provided current research findings and presented written information to Mr. Reynolds to read about current treatment of HIV seroconversion and AIDS.

Mr. and Mrs. Reynolds' questions were answered honestly, their concerns were discussed openly, and factors which may have affected Mr. Reynolds' initial appraisal of his situation were identified. By the conclusion of counseling during week one, Mr. Reynolds verbalized that he had a thorough understanding of his disease process and knew where to obtain additional information about it. Mr. Reynolds was also able to identify factors which affected his initial appraisal of his illness. He realized that his personal beliefs about HIV seroconversion and AIDS, his commitment to a health-promoting lifestyle, and his strong religious beliefs had affected his initial appraisal of his illness. Additionally, he recognized that the unexpectedness of the diagnosis, uncertainty of the disease process, and ambiguity about prognosis impacted his initial appraisal of the illness.

During the second week of counseling, Mr. Reynolds and Ms. Miller identified areas of the illness that Mr. Reynolds could control, such as diet, exercise regime, sexual intercourse practices, maintenance of a health-promoting lifestyle, and disclosure of his illness. Ms. Miller encouraged Mr. Reynolds to use problem-solving methods to decide how to control these areas. By the end of the second week of counseling, Mr. Reynolds was able to use problem-solving methods to plan a family meeting to tell his children of his illness. He also understood the necessity of having Mrs. Reynolds tested. He suggested to his family that his children and grandchildren also be tested.

During the third week of counseling, Mr. Reynolds and Ms. Miller identified factors affecting his coping process. Those factors which impeded the process were identified and modified. Mr. and Mrs. Reynolds reviewed their initial beliefs and fears about AIDS and realized that they had some misconceptions about the illness. They discussed the social stigma associated with the diagnosis and agreed that their community service activities would focus on public education about the disease. They recognized that such a diagnosis is very threatening, but that some areas of it can be controlled.

Those factors which facilitated the coping process were identified and used. The Reynolds recognized that John's asymptomatic state could best be maintained by continuing to follow a health-promoting lifestyle. They identified their strong religious beliefs as major resources for coping with the illness. They recounted past evidence of effective use of problem-solving skills in dealing with stress. They listed social skills which could assist them with coping. They identified their children, their minister, and the community AIDS clinic as social supports which could help them cope. They recognized that they are financially secure; if John should need to retire early, they would not have to worry about money.

During the fourth week of counseling Mr. and Mrs. Reynolds were able to openly discuss the illness without anger. They had told their children about the diagnosis and had received support from them. Mary had been tested for the virus and was currently HIV negative. They viewed as challenging the ability to keep John in an asymptomatic state. They were using problem-focused coping processes to deal with the diagnosis.

The Reynolds and Ms. Miller agreed to terminate biweekly counseling sessions at this time. Mr. Reynolds stated that, although he still felt stress about his illness, the amount of stress had decreased significantly and was now manageable. Ms. Miller encouraged the Reynolds to become actively involved in group counseling through the AIDS clinic. She also reminded the Reynolds that the individual counseling sessions could resume any time the Reynolds felt the need for them.

Evaluating

Product Evaluation (Extent the Goal(s) and Predicted Outcomes were Met)

1. By the end of the fourth week of counseling Mr. Reynolds was able to discuss his HIV seroconversion without indignation, anger, or denial.
2. Mr. Reynolds expressed a significant decrease in the amount of stress he felt about the illness.

Process Evaluation

Nurse Focus (extent that planned nursing interventions were implemented).
1. The nurse decreased ambiguity about the disease process by providing written and oral information about HIV seroconversion and AIDS.
2. The nurse assisted the Reynolds to identify parts of the disease process which could be controlled.
3. The nurse identified personal and situational factors which affected Mr. Reynolds' initial appraisal of the illness.
4. The nurse refocused Mr. Reynolds' energy toward problem-solving.
5. The nurse helped Mr. Reynolds to identify and modify constraints against coping and to identify and use resources which facilitated coping with the illness.

Client Focus (extent that the etiology component of the nursing diagnosis statement was modified).
1. Mr. Reynolds identified and used effective methods of coping which resulted in stress reduction.

2. Mr. Reynolds identified coping resources to assist him in coping with the stress.
3. Mr. Reynolds identified constraints that impeded him from coping with the stress.
4. Mr. Reynolds redirected his emotion-focused coping response into a problem-focused coping response.
5. Mr. Reynolds reappraised his illness as challenging instead of threatening.

SUMMARY

This section described and applied Lazarus' coping theory in the context of the nursing process to a client case. The theory was used to demonstrate how a nurse might assist a client cope with the stress of HIV seroconversion.

REFERENCES

Folkman, S., Lazarus, R. S., Dunkel-Schetter, C., DeLongis, A., & Gruen, R. J. (1986). Dynamics of a stressful encounter: Cognitive appraisal, coping, and encounter outcomes. *Journal of Personality and Social Psychology, 50,* 992–1003.

Jalowiec, A., & Powers, M. J. (1981). Stress and coping in hypertensive and emergency room patients. *Nursing Research, 30,* 10–15.

Kirschling, J. M., & McBride, A. B. (1989). Effects of age and sex on the experience of widowhood. *Western Journal of Nursing Research, 11,* 207–218.

Kobasa, S. C. (1979). Stressful life event, personality, and health: An inquiry into hardiness. *Journal of Personality and Social Psychology, 37,* 1–11.

Lazarus, R. S. (1976). *Patterns of adjustment* (3rd. ed.). New York: McGraw-Hill.

Lazarus, R. S., & Folkman, S. (1984). *Stress, appraisal and coping.* New York: Springer Publishing Co.

Mishel, M. H. (1990). Reconceptualization of the uncertainty in illness theory. *Image, 22,* 256–261.

Mishel, M. H. (1988). Uncertainty in illness. *Image, 20,* 225–232.

Nyamathi, A. (1989). Comprehensive health seeking and coping paradigm. *Journal of Advanced Nursing, 14,* 281–290.

Pollock, S. E. (1989). Adaptive responses to diabetes mellitus. *Western Journal of Nursing Research, 11,* 265–275.

SUGGESTED READINGS

Kobasa, S. C. (1979). Stressful life events, personality, and health: An inquiry into hardiness. *Journal of Personality and Social Psychology, 37,* 1–11.

Mishel, M. H. (1981). The measurement of uncertainty in illness. *Nursing Research, 30,* 258–263.

Mishel, M. H. (1984). Perceived uncertainty and stress in illness. *Research in Nursing and Health, 7,* 163–171.

Mishel, M. H. (1988). Uncertainty in illness. *Image, 20,* 225–232.

Mishel, M. H., & Braden, C. J. (1988). Finding meaning: Antecedents of uncertainty. *Nursing Research, 37,* 98–103.

O'Connor, P. C. (1989). *The hardiness for health professionals scale: A design and validation study.* Unpublished doctoral dissertation. Temple University.

Rich, V. L., & Rich, A. R. (1987). Personality hardiness and burnout in female staff nurses. *Image, 19,* 63–66.

Chapter 8

Peplau's Theory with an Emphasis on Anxiety

Wilda K. Arnold and Rose Nieswiadomy

Anxiety is a universal emotion. This emotion may be manifested either overtly or covertly, but is present to some degree in many clients seen by nurses. When anxiety is high, the client exhibits dysfunctional behavior. The case history of Randall Morrison will demonstrate how Peplau's theory can be used by the nurse to help clients learn to reduce anxiety to a level that promotes adaptive behavior.

CLIENT CASE

Randall Morrison is a 38-year-old male who is a professional singer. He visited his family physician, complaining of diarrhea. A physical examination revealed that he was physically healthy. The doctor prescribed Lomotil 2 mg. to be taken after each bowel movement.

Two weeks later Mr. Morrison came back to see the doctor, stating that the diarrhea had not stopped. He had lost 3 pounds since his last visit. Further examinations (gastrointestinal series and a barium enema) showed results to be within normal limits. In talking with the doctor, Mr. Morrison stated, "My nerves are really bad." He expressed concern about his career and the demands it made on him. He said, "I get tense just before a performance."

Mrs. Morrison pointed out that her husband's diarrhea seemed to occur on the days he was scheduled to perform. She also reported that her husband does not believe he is singing as well as he should be able to sing. The physician prescribed Valium 5 mg. twice daily.

A week later Mr. Morrison's wife called the doctor and reported that her husband had become "very upset" the night before and had to cancel a singing engagement. About an hour before the performance he had started having diarrhea, perspiring profusely, and complained "I feel like I'm choking." During the previous week he had been unable to remember the words of songs and had to be prompted several times. The physician suggested that Mr. Morrison be seen by a nurse who had experience working with patients with similar problems.

Mrs. Morrison called the nurse the next day, stating that her husband needed to see someone as soon as possible. She reported that he had been unable to sleep the night before and that the Valium had not relieved the symptoms. An appointment was made for Mr. Morrison to see the nurse that afternoon.

During the intake interview the nurse noted that Mr. Morrison was perspiring, fidgeted in the chair, and had difficulty expressing his thoughts and answering questions. He stated, "I feel like I'm choking and this diarrhea is making me weak."

Mr. Morrison reported that he had begun singing as a teenager and always got a "little uptight" just before a performance. These feelings had progressively gotten worse over the past 2 years. When asked what happened 2 years ago, he stated, "not anything that I can recall. It's just that so many singers I know begin to have problems with their vocal cords, which makes it difficult to sing. I just don't want that to happen to me. I don't want to be a 'has been.' I've let my family down. They really depended on me and thought I'd be a great singer. It seems I've just been average. I've never made the big time like I kept thinking I would." His singing engagements had become less frequent and his agent reported that it was more difficult to secure bookings.

PATTERNING CUES FROM CLIENT CASE

The nurse interviewed Mr. Morrison for the purpose of gathering data about his presenting problem. He said that the diarrhea and choking sensation were his main problems. When the nurse began to ask questions, it became apparent that his major concern was the difficulty he was having related to his singing performances. It is important that both verbal and nonverbal cues be included in the data. Based upon the information Mr. Morrison provided, the nurse concluded that his difficulty in performing singing engagements was a manifestation of anxiety. There are a number of indicators, both verbal and nonverbal, which helped the nurse identify anxiety:

1. Physiological symptoms indicative of anxiety, such as diarrhea, perspiring, and choking sensation for which no physical cause was determined during medical examination.
2. Cognitive clues, such as difficulty concentrating, expressing his thoughts and answering questions, and remembering words to songs.
3. Tense feelings prior to singing performance that have become progressively worse over the past 2 years and that are now interfering with his performances.
4. Subjective report, "My nerves are really bad."

The nurse will observe Mr. Morrison, noting relations and connections in the data he provides. She will consider the data and the theories that might apply to this client's situation. She will then select a theory that best explains what she is seeing and hearing and that will be the most beneficial in helping her to analyze the data. This theory will then guide the plan of care for Mr. Morrison.

SELECTED RELEVANT THEORIES

A number of theories address the concept of anxiety and could provide direction for the nurse when caring for a client who is anxious. Three of these theories will be discussed in order to demonstrate how each theory explains the origin of anxiety and to show how each of the three provides guidelines for interventions. The theories of Rollo May and Karen Horney will be presented briefly; then a more detailed discussion of Hildegard Peplau's theory, with an emphasis on anxiety, will be presented. Peplau's theory will be used to develop a nursing care plan for Randall Morrison.

May's Existential Theory

May's (1977) theory of existentialism is concerned with the individual as a human who is becoming and who is emerging into the future. The theory is concerned with a person's subjective awareness of his or her existence. A person is always moving into the future. Responsibility for and awareness of self are characteristics a human being must possess in order to become self-actualized.

One of the major concepts of existentialism, which has application for this case study, is that of anxiety. May (1977) defined anxiety as "the apprehension cued off by a threat to some value that the individual holds essential to his existence as a personality" (p. 205). Anxiety is the most painful threat a human being can experience because it is a threat to the loss of the existence of the self (May, Angel, & Ellenberger, 1958).

May (1977) differentiated normal from neurotic anxiety. Normal anxiety is characterized by the recognition and realistic appraisal of threats that an individual experiences. The individual confronts these situations directly and solves the problems caused by the threats. Neurotic anxiety occurs when there is an incapacity for coping with threats. This incapacity is due to inner psychological patterns that keep the person from using his or her powers to solve problems.

Because anxiety is a response to the threat to essential values, which are considered necessary for the person's existence, May (1977) contended that security patterns that exist between the infant and his or her parents are the essential values for the infant. Thus, neurosis, or the inability to confront anxiety constructively, has its origin in childhood. May further stated that neurosis occurs as the result of the child not being able to solve threatening interpersonal problems.

Existential psychotherapy is considered a long-term treatment approach and is based "on an understanding of what makes man the human being" (May et al., 1958, p. 35). The central process of existential psychotherapy is to assist the individual to recognize and experience his or her own existence (May et al., 1958). One of the first steps in the psychotherapeutic process is to help the client know anxiety and to accept it as an inevitable part of human life (May, 1977).

There are two approaches that may be used in helping an individual resolve the problems associated with anxiety. The first approach involves an expansion of awareness and the second involves reeducation. In the former the individual identifies what values are being threatened and then becomes conscious of conflicts between his or her goals and how these conflicts developed. In the latter, the individual restructures his or her goals, makes decisions, and moves toward implementing these decisions in a responsible manner (May, 1977).

A nursing diagnosis for Mr. Morrison, generated from this theory, is "incapacitating anxiety prior to singing performances related to threat to essential values." When Mr. Morrison considered the possibility of failure in performances, he felt a threat to something he valued. He was faced with destruction of his existence (May, 1977). The nurse would first help Mr. Morrison to reduce his anxiety to normal limits. The next step would be to help him increase his awareness of the anxious feelings and to understand them as a normal part of his life (May, 1977). As the nurse and client continue to work together, the nurse would assist Mr. Morrison to either expand his awareness of the threats and conflicts he is experiencing or help him redefine career goals and support him as he learns to make decisions in a responsible manner. Additionally, the nurse would help Mr. Morrison to develop relationships with others.

Horney's Theory

Horney (1937) proposed that anxiety may be an important factor in a person's life without the person being aware of it. She stated, "One may have more anxiety than one is aware of or may have anxiety without being aware of it at all" (p. 58). She contended that a great deal of anxiety is caused by our culture and that it is at the core of neurosis. Horney (1937) wrote that although experiences in childhood provide conditions for neuroses, they are not the only factors that cause difficulties. She maintained that anxiety can occur any time stress is present.

Anxiety is an emotional reaction to a hidden and subjective danger. This anxiety is disproportionate to the situation. It is a feeling of "being small, insignificant, helpless, deserted, endangered, in a world that is out to abuse, cheat, attack, humiliate, betray, envy" (Horney, 1937, p. 92). There is a feeling of great danger and a sense of being defenseless against it. These feelings are caused by intrapsychic factors and will influence the individual's attitude toward self and others. These influences may be observed as emotional isolation, along with a decrease in self-confidence. There is a conflict between the desire to depend on others and the inability to do so because of distrust toward them.

Horney (1937) maintained that anxiety is the center of neurosis. She defined neurosis as "a psychic disturbance brought about by fears and defenses against these fears and by attempts to find compromise solutions for conflicting tendencies" (pp. 28–29). All neuroses have two characteristics. One of these is a rigidity in reaction, and the other is a discrepancy between potentialities and accomplishments.

Although an individual may be able to engage in usual activities, if there is anxiety related to them, the manner in which the person functions will be altered. For example, when engaging in an activity which arouses anxiety, the individual may feel an undue amount of fatigue or strain, there may be an impairment in carrying out the activity, or the pleasure of the activity may be decreased.

Horney (1937) wrote that anxiety is one of the most tormenting emotions individuals can experience and that people will go to any lengths to avoid feeling anxious. She identified three elements of anxiety which make it so tormenting—feelings of helplessness, irrationality, and the belief that something is wrong within oneself.

People use four main means of escaping anxiety. The first method is that of rationalization, or the turning of anxiety into rational fear and then shifting the responsibility for it outside oneself. The second method of escaping anxiety is that of denial, which excludes the anxiety from conscious awareness. Another way of handling anxiety is to anesthetize or narcotize it. This may be done in a number of ways, such as by using drugs or by becoming a workaholic. Finally, all situations causing anxiety may be avoided, either consciously or unconsciously (Horney, 1937). Psychotherapy is oriented to the here-and-now and aims to find the meaning that certain situations have for the individual (Horney, 1937). The client is helped to set both long-term and short-term goals, to face the real self, release potential, and adapt to the culture (Murray & Huelskoetter, 1991).

The nursing diagnosis for Mr. Morrison, generated from Horney's theory, is "overwhelming anxiety prior to singing performances related to feelings of being defenseless against perceived danger." Nursing interventions would help Mr. Morrison to examine the meaning of his singing, especially those situations that precipitate his anxiety. The nurse would help him to set both long-term and short-term goals and to examine discrepancies between his abilities and accomplishments and his perceptions of his potentialities. Mr. Morrison would also be assisted to become aware of the conflicts he is experiencing, of which he is unaware.

Peplau's Theory

The theory of Peplau (1952) is based on interpersonal relationships. Peplau described this theory as providing a dynamic orientation to the understanding of human behavior. She stated that the theory uses principles from the biological, psychological, and social sciences and explains the meaning of interactions among people in a situation. A number of individuals influenced Peplau's thinking and work. One of these individuals was Harry Stack Sullivan. Many of the tenets of Sullivanian theory (1953) are found in Peplau's work.

Peplau's theory includes a number of concepts that are useful in guiding nursing practice. It is beyond the scope of this chapter to include all of these concepts. Therefore, only those most relevant to the case study presented will be discussed. The major emphasis will be on anxiety.

DESCRIPTION OF PEPLAU'S THEORY WITH AN EMPHASIS ON ANXIETY

The central focus of Peplau's theory concerns the interactions that occur among individuals in a given situation. It is within the context of these interactions, or relationships, that behavior occurs. When these relationships are disturbed and human needs cannot be met, emotions such as tension, anxiety, and frustration are often felt. Needs are both physiological and psychological and generate tension. The tension generated by needs creates energy that is changed into behavior. Peplau (1952) wrote that "all behavior aims to reduce tension arising from needs" (p. 80). When a need is not met, not only is tension generated, but more mature needs cannot emerge. Or, if the need is blocked before satisfaction of these urges has been experienced, frustration occurs. This frustration may constitute a threat to the personality (Peplau, 1952).

Peplau stressed the relationship between behavior and the tension generated by unmet needs. She maintained that "all human behavior is purposeful and goal seeking in terms of satisfaction and/or security" (1952, p. 86). When a need is strong, all behavior is directed toward fulfilling that need and, as a result, other needs may not be noticed. The individual behaves, either wittingly or unwittingly, in terms of his or her perception of self as it relates to others. The skills a person brings into play when his or her personality is threatened also help determine behavior.

Peplau (1952) emphasized the importance of the nurse-patient relationship in nursing. She maintained that nursing practice occurs within a relationship between a client and a nurse and that the main work goes on during this interactive process. The crucial elements in a nursing situation are the client and the nurse, as well as the interaction that occurs between them.

Peplau (1987) proposed that the aim of the nurse is to assess the interpersonal interactions that take place between a client and others, which would help in the identification of those human responses and patterns that are problematic. Included in this assessment would be not only listening to the facts the client presents, but also observing gestures and body movements. Interventions would focus upon establishing and maintaining a goal-oriented relationship with the client (Peplau, 1987). All nurse-patient contacts provide opportunities for the nurse to come to know that client as a human being who is having difficulties and to help that person stretch his or her capabilities.

Major Concepts

The concepts selected from Peplau's theory (Table 8.1) that have relevancy for the case of Mr. Morrison are:

1. self (self-system)
2. unmet expectations perceived as a threat to self-system
3. anxiety
4. behavioral responses to anxiety

Table 8.1   Major concepts of Peplau's theory with an emphasis on anxiety

Self-system
  Self-views
  Self-image
  Self-worth
  Self-esteem
Unmet expectations perceived as threat to self-system
Anxiety
  Mild (1+)
  Moderate (2+)
  Severe (3+)
  Panic (4+)
Behavioral Responses to Anxiety
  "Acting out"
  Somatizing
  "Freezing-on-the-spot"
  Using anxiety in the service of learning

Theoretical Definitions of Major Concepts

Self (Self-System)

Peplau (1990) defined the self as "an abstraction; it is a convenient way of describing a function of the total person" (p. 107). The self, or self-system, is revised during interpersonal relationships throughout life. Peplau compared the self to a theoretical framework in that it "serves as an organizing structure through which experiences, events, and people are perceived and known, accepted, or rejected" (p. 107).

Peplau (1990) indicated that the self is a system composed of self-views, self-image, self-worth, and self-esteem.

1) *Self-views* are conceptions of oneself made up of baseline reflected appraisals from caretakers in early life and the incremental additions obtained from the individual's subsequent experiences.

2) *Self-image* is the ideal picture of oneself which is conveyed to the world. It portrays how one wishes to be seen by others and may not be congruent with the self-view.

3) *Self-worth* is a by-product of a close interpersonal relationship with a best friend. This relationship provides validation, from outside the family, of one's personal worth. The evaluation of oneself and of one's abilities are also included in this part of the self-system.

4) *Self-esteem* includes the confidence an individual has in his or her abilities and which serves as a measure of self-praise.

Unmet Expectations Perceived as a Threat to Self-System

"Expectations" is a term used by Peplau to indicate a general classification that includes such cognitions as "assumptions, preconceptions, attributions, wishes, wants, beliefs, values, hopes, desires, needs, goals, self-views and the like" (Peplau, 1990, p. 96). According to Peplau (1990) expectations are either personal, situational, sociocultural, or a mixture of these types. Peplau (1952, 1990) explained that in anxiety an expectation becomes operative (up front in the mind) but the expectation is not met. This unmet expectation is considered a threat to the self and requires an immediate behavioral response in order to restore comfort. Thus a person's expectations may be unmet at any given time. If this unmet expectation is interpreted as a threat to the security of the individual, anxiety occurs.

Anxiety

Anxiety is "a response to unknown danger that is felt, experienced as discomfort, and that arms the human organism for mobilizing resources to meet the difficulty" (Peplau, 1952, p. 127). This behavioral response can be either in the direction of adaptation, learning, and personal growth or in the direction of maladaptation and illness (Peplau, 1990).

Anxiety provides the organism with the stimulus for mobilizing resources to face the problem. Therefore, it can be thought of as the first step in problem solving because the individual has a felt need and concentrates all resources on meeting that need (Peplau, 1952).

Anxiety occurs on a continuum and can be categorized as mild, moderate, severe, or panic anxiety.

1) *Mild Anxiety (1+)*—alertness is increased, connections can be seen, the processes of learning are operative, and problem solving can occur.
2) *Moderate Anxiety (2+)*—the perceptual field narrows, selective inattention (failure to notice aspects of an experience) occurs.
3) *Severe Anxiety (3+)*—the perceptual field is reduced (focus is on detail or scattered details); the view of the problem is greatly narrowed, with selective inattention.
4) *Panic Anxiety (4+)*—feelings of terror, details are "blown up," there is an inability to test reality, and behavior is directed toward obtaining relief (Peplau, 1952, 1963).

Behavioral Responses to Anxiety

Four major behavioral patterns (Peplau, 1963) are used to transform the energy of anxiety: "acting out," somatizing, "freezing-on-the-spot," and using anxiety in the service of learning.

1) *"Acting out"*—behavior may be overt, such as being angry, or covert, such as feeling resentment.
2) *Somatizing*—evidenced by psychosomatic complaints.
3) *"Freezing-on-the-spot"*—manifested by withdrawal.
4) *Using anxiety in the service of learning*—seen when an individual can use all the processes involved in learning to acquire knowledge or a skill.

Examples of Concepts Relevant to Clinical Practice

Peplau's theory provides the nurse with a number of concepts useful in nursing practice. The two concepts relevant for all nurses in all areas of nursing practice are those of anxiety and the self-system. Clinical examples of these concepts will be discussed.

Self-System

Jonathan, a 19-year-old truck driver, has received three tickets for traffic violations in the past month and has, consequently, been fired from his job. He views these events as further rejections and as a failure on his part. He reports being rejected by his mother and father after their divorce when he was 5 years old. He was sent to live with his grandparents. Family members were very verbal about his inability to make friends or attain good grades.

The recurring negative appraisals Jonathan has received from significant others, coupled with his appraisal of failure, have been incorporated into his self-system, giving him a negative self-view.

Anxiety

Joan is a 19-year-old college freshman, referred to the school counselor by her academic advisor. Two hours prior to taking her first college examination, Joan had called the professor stating she would be unable to take the test because of a "migraine headache." Each time the professor scheduled a time for Joan to take the test, she would call complaining of headaches, abdominal cramping, and nausea. Joan is evidencing physical signs of severe anxiety and the relief behavior of somatizing.

Major Relational Statements

The concepts in Peplau's theory can be joined in relational statements. These relational statements then depict the progression of events that result in behaviors indicative of anxiety.

As a result of interactions with others, a self-system develops. The self-system serves as an anti-anxiety system, which evolves and changes as interpersonal relations are developed. Behaviors evolve within the context of interpersonal relations. When an unmet expectation occurs that is considered as a threat to the self (threat to the security of the individual), anxiety occurs. The energy of anxiety is converted into behaviors that may be health-promoting or illness-producing. If anxiety becomes severe, behaviors will be in the direction of illness. The greater the anxiety, the more dysfunctional is the behavior. If anxiety is reduced, psychological growth is more apt to occur. Individuals can learn to recognize the events that precipitate their anxiety and subsequent relief behavior.

IMPLICATIONS OF PEPLAU'S THEORY
FOR NURSING PRACTICE

This section will discuss anxiety as described by Peplau (1952, 1963, 1979, 1989a, 1989b, 1990) in nursing practice with an individual client. Assessment factors, methods of assessing, theory-specific diagnoses, the nursing care plan, and evaluation of the nursing care plan will be included.

Factors to be Assessed and Methods of Assessment

The data collected by the nurse will help him or her to understand the situation that precipitated the anxiety in the client, as well as assist in the identification of the client's level of anxiety. The client's way of handling the anxiety, how the anxiety is manifested, and what causes the anxiety to escalate are additional assessment data to be obtained. Peplau (1979) stated, "Because anxiety is an energy it cannot be studied directly. Rather it must be studied through its transformation into effects or behavior" (p. 17). Therefore, the nurse's assessment of the client will be based on behaviors exhibited by the client.

Assessment data are collected through verbal interactions with the client. Data may also be collected from significant others. Additional methods of assessing are direct observation of the client's verbal and nonverbal behaviors as well as patterns of interaction with the nurse and others. Examples of assessment data relating to anxiety and the theoretical basis for the needed information will be presented.

Assessment Data

1. Description of situation precipitating symptoms
   A. Nonverbal clues as situation is described
   B. Who was present
   C. Action taken
   D. How long situation lasted
   E. Expectation not met

Theoretical Basis

"Look for obvious physical symptoms . . . Listen to subjective complaints, fears, dreams, and worries. Look for non-verbal clues concerning feelings . . . Get as much information as you can" (Murray & Huelskoeter, 1991, p. 425).

"Constructive learning takes place when the patient can perceive and focus on crucial cues in the situation, through his own efforts, and when he can develop responses to them independently of the nurse" (Peplau, 1952, p. 35).

2. Present level of anxiety
   A. Subjective description of feelings, fears, concerns
   B. Communication
      1. speech pattern
      2. affect
      3. verbal behavior
      4. nonverbal behavior

"The words are important, but also note how the words are stated" (Murray & Huelskoetter, 1991, p. 425).

5. hesitation
6. pitch of voice
3. Previous experience with similar situations
   A. How handled
   B. Outcome

4. Situations escalating anxiety
   A. When
   B. Where
   C. Feelings before increase in anxiety
5. Cognitive Abilities
   A. Reality testing
   B. Problem solving
   C. Thought processes
6. Physiological manifestations
   A. Tachycardia
   B. Palpitations
   C. Tremors
   D. Muscle tension
   E. Diarrhea
   F. Frequent urination
   H. Cold clammy skin
   I. Dilated pupils
   J. Pallor
   K. Changes in eating habits
   L. Restlessness
   M. Other
7. Psychological manifestations
   A. Tension
   B. Apprehension
   C. Indecisiveness
   D. Oversensitivity
   E. Tearfulness
   F. Agitation
   G. Irritability
   H. Dread
   I. Panic

"As anxiety increases . . . ability to observe what is happening and to make use of past experiences in evaluating present events gives way to overfocalization on the discomfort" (Peplau, 1952, p. 128).

"The aim is to get the patient to describe what it was that he had in mind or thought, or wished, or wanted, or sought or expected" (Peplau, 1979, p. 21).

"Another area in which there are observable effects has to do with the thought processes" (Peplau, 1979, p. 18).

"Anxiety triggers an immediate physiological reaction" (Peplau, 1990, p. 94). "The discomfort of anxiety is felt in some body part . . . The extent of the discomfort is dependent on the degree of anxiety" (Peplau, 1990, p. 97). "Where the discomfort is felt can only be determined by asking the patient" (Peplau, 1990, p. 99). "The effects of anxiety can be noticed in terms of motor behavior" (Peplau, 1979, p. 18).

"There is an awareness of apprehension, felt discomfort, and physiological reactions" (Peplau, 1990, p. 94).

J. Powerlessness
K. Decrease of self-worth

8. Relief Behaviors
   A. Patterns of behavior
   B. Sequence of behaviors
   C. Types of behaviors
      1. acting out
      2. somatizing
      3. freezing on spot
      4. using anxiety to foster learning

"There are four major behavioral patterns used to transform the energy of anxiety" (Peplau, 1963, p. 327).

9. Degree of anxiety
   A. Mild
   B. Moderate
   C. Severe
   D. Panic

"The nurse must be able to distinguish presence of these varying degrees of anxiety for interventions are based on discrimination of the degree of anxiety" (Peplau, 1989a, p. 52).

10. Nurse's feelings and level of anxiety

"Reduction of anxiety and bringing about constructive changes in the patient often require examination of how the nurse feels about the patient . . ." (Peplau, 1952, p. 157).
"Your only clue to your client's anxiety may be your own feelings" (Murray & Huelskoetter, 1991, p. 425).

Theory-Specific Diagnoses

Peplau (1989b) asserted that nurses diagnose and treat "those human responses of clients in relation to psychosocial or psychiatric problems, that detract from and prevent healthy living in the community" (p. 193). She also told nurses: "You need to think in terms of where you can bring about change, where you can be the agent of change in behalf of the client" (Peplau, 1979, p. 21).

Response Component

The response component of the nursing diagnosis is anxiety. The anxiety is manifested in some specific behaviors. Therefore, the response component of the nursing diagnosis statement may be stated as anxiety or a more specific behavior such as:

1. Potential to harm self or others.
2. Decrease in problem-solving abilities.
3. Physiological disturbances.
4. Obsessive behavior (repetitive thoughts).
5. Compulsive behavior (handwashing).
6. Phobic behavior (fear of flying).

Etiology Component

The etiology component of the nursing diagnosis concerns an unmet expectation regarding the self-system. This unmet expectation is interpreted as a threat to the security of the individual.

1. Unmet expectations concerning image of self as parent.
2. Unmet expectations concerning image of self as family provider.
3. Unmet expectations concerning image of one's job performance.

Nursing Diagnosis

Examples of nursing diagnoses generated from Peplau's theory would be:

1. "Potential for harm to self (4+ anxiety) related to unmet expectation concerning image of one's academic performance."
2. "GI disturbances each morning before going to work (3+ anxiety) related to unmet expectation concerning image of one's job performance."

Nursing Care Plan

Following the formulation of the nursing diagnosis, the care plan will be developed, with goals and intervention techniques based on Peplau's theory. Because the nurse often encounters an anxious client, Peplau developed specific interventions for anxiety. Plans will include strategies to help the client reduce anxiety. These plans and the goals would be made conjointly by the client and the nurse. In order for a reduction in the level of the client's anxiety to occur, the person must be assisted to undergo a self-examination of the anxiety.

The nurse-patient relationship will provide the nurse and client an opportunity to determine what each wants and expects from the relationship. Peplau (1952) wrote: "keeping anxiety within tolerable limits and making use of the energy it provides are nursing functions that require understanding of what is happening in the relationships" (p. 157).

Because anxiety is communicated interpersonally, the nurse monitors his or her own level of anxiety. Peplau (1990) wrote that "anxiety can also be triggered when a person feels the anxiety another person in the same situation is then experiencing" (p. 94).

Implementation of the Care Plan

Documentation of the nursing actions carried out will be recorded by the nurse in a detailed and precise manner. Peplau (1952), in writing about recording, said, "the exact wording is more important than abbreviated or cryptic recording of the complaint" (p. 307). The client's record will reveal the extent to which the care plan was implemented and the degree of change that occurred in the client.

Evaluation of the Care Plan

Product evaluation will be determined by comparing predicted outcomes to the actual outcomes. Product evaluation for Mr. Morrison will be measured by the degree of anxiety reduction (response component of the nursing diagnosis). Process evaluation will be evaluated by determining the extent to which the nursing actions were actually carried out and by determining if the client is now able to deal with the events(s) perceived to be a threat to the security of self (change in the etiology component of the nursing diagnosis).

THEORY-DIRECTED NURSING CARE
FOR THE MORRISON CASE

The use of Peplau's theory in working with the client in the clinical case vignette will now be discussed. The use of the various steps of the nursing process model (Ziegler, Vaughan-Wrobel, & Erlen, 1986) for the clinical case will be demonstrated.

Assessing

The information contained in the case study is organized under the categories directing assessing.

1. *Description of situation-precipitating symptoms*—He does not believe he is singing as well as he has in the past. He expresses concern that many singers have problems with their vocal cords; he does not want that to happen to him. He does not want to be a "has been." He feels he has let his family down as they expected that he would be a great singer; he believes that perhaps he is only average.

2. *Present level of anxiety*—His wife says he needs to be seen by someone immediately; he is unable to sleep and symptoms are escalating.

3. *Previous experience with similar situations*—He always got a little uptight just before a performance. His feelings have become progressively worse over the past 2 years.

4. *Situations escalating anxiety*—"I get tense just before a performance." Diarrhea occurs on the days he is scheduled to perform. He became very upset and had to cancel a singing engagement.

5. *Cognitive abilities*—He is having difficulty concentrating, expressing his thoughts, answering questions, and he is forgetting words to songs.

6. *Physiological manifestations*—He is experiencing diarrhea with negative findings on physical examination. He has lost 3 pounds, is perspiring, complains of a choking sensation, and is unable to sleep.
7. *Psychological manifestations*—"My nerves are really bad."
8. *Relief behaviors*—diarrhea (somatizing) and canceled engagement (freezing-on-the spot).
9. *Degree of anxiety*—Severe to panic. His behavior is directed toward obtaining relief.
10. *Nurse's feelings and level of anxiety*—No data in case presentation.

Mr. Morrison's behaviors indicate that his anxiety is interfering with his career. From the data in the vignette it is evident that his symptoms are escalating and he is becoming more incapacitated.

Diagnosing

Based on the data presented in the client case the following nursing diagnosis was formulated.

3+ Anxiety Prior to Singing Performances Related to Unmet Expectations Concerning Image of Self as a Professional Singer

Response: 3+ anxiety prior to singing performances

Subjective Data	Objective Data
"I get tense before a performance."	
" I feel like I'm choking."	Has had to cancel a singing engagement.
"This diarrhea is making me weak."	Wife reported husband had become "very upset" and was unable to remember words of songs.
"My nerves are really bad."	

Etiology: unmet expectations concerning image of self as a professional singer

Subjective Data	Objective Data
"I've let my family down; they depended on me."	Wife stated, "He doesn't think he is singing as well as he should be."
"I've never made the big time like I thought I would."	Singing engagements are becoming fewer.

Planning

Goals and predicted outcomes are formulated based on the subjective and objective data of the response component of the nursing diagnosis (3+ anxiety prior to singing performances).

Goals:
Mr. Morrison will:

1. Report fewer physiological symptoms of anxiety.
2. Be able to resume his singing engagements without feelings of tenseness and choking.

Predicted Outcomes:
After 2 weeks, Mr. Morrison will:

1. Report only occasional episodes of diarrhea.
2. Report no choking sensations prior to singing, but will still have occasional moderate tenseness.
3. Keep all singing engagements.
4. Require only occasional prompting during performances.

After one month, Mr. Morrison will:

1. Report no episodes of diarrhea in the previous week.
2. Report occasional mild tenseness.
3. Perform with assurance and confidence, without prompting.

Nursing Interventions:
Nursing interventions and the rationale for these actions are formulated based on the etiology component of the nursing diagnosis statement (unmet expectations concerning image of self as a professional singer).

1. Establish a nurse-patient relationship that will enable Mr. Morrison to identify behavioral cues of anxiety and the events which preceded development of anxiety.
2. Reduce anxiety to a level where learning can occur.
3. Assist the client to understand the dynamics of anxiety.
4. Teach the client methods of recognizing and relieving anxiety.
5. Teach the client the relationship between his behaviors and his unmet expectations.
6. Examine own anxiety in interactions with client.
7. Help client to compare his expectations of self against realistic expectations.
8. Help client verbalize the threat to his security that his singing career generates.
9. Help client to plan realistic career goals for the future.

The nursing actions that will be presented are in a continuous list. However, in intervening with Mr. Morrison, certain nursing actions would occur in the first session, while other actions would be carried out in subsequent sessions. Nursing actions would be determined by the progress being made by the client.

Nursing Actions

1. Initiate, establish, and maintain a nurse-patient relationship by using warmth and respect.

2. Praise Mr. Morrison for seeking help.

3. Monitor the degree of Mr. Morrison's anxiety on an ongoing basis.

Rationale

". . .the main work goes on in an interactive process during which the participants are a nurse and a patient" (Peplau, 1987, p. 201).

"Seeking assistance on the basis of a need felt but poorly understood, is often the first step in a dynamic learning experience from which a constructive next step in personality growth can occur" (Peplau, 1952, p. 19).

"The nurse must be able to distinguish the presence of these varying degrees of anxiety for interventions are based on discrimination of the degree of anxiety" (Peplau, 1989a, p. 52).

4. Maintain a calm environment and approach in sessions with Mr. Morrison.

"Anxiety can also be triggered when a person feels the anxiety another person in the same situation is then experiencing; this transmission occurs by way of empathic observation, the ability to feel in oneself the emotions of another person during an interpersonal relationship" (Peplau, 1990, p. 94).

5. Examine own feelings and reactions to client.

"Reduction of anxiety and bringing about constructive changes in the patient often requires examination of how the nurse feels about the patient" (Peplau, 1952, p. 157).

6. Observe the behavior Mr. Morrison exhibits when anxious and what he does to relieve the discomfort. Ask him if he is feeling anxious or uncomfortable.

"What you are trying to do is to get the individual to recognize the underlying phenomena related to the relief behavior that he is using" (Peplau, 1979, p. 20).

7. Encourage Mr. Morrison to describe what happens just before he goes on stage to sing and what he thought would happen if he went onstage and began to sing.

". . . help the patient to formulate what it was that he had in mind, or thought, or wanted, or sought, or expected . . ." (Peplau, 1979, p. 21).

8. Assist Mr. Morrison to connect anxiety to its relief behavior by asking him what he does to get more comfortable when he feels tense.

"When the client is able to make connections . . . he is already beginning to see relationships" (Peplau, 1979, p. 20).

9. Ask if the choking feeling decreases once he decides not to sing.

"All behavior is purposeful and goal seeking in terms of satisfaction and/ or security" (Peplau, 1952, p. 86).

10. Help Mr. Morrison to verbalize what he hoped would happen during his singing career and what he perceives has happened.

"Get the operative expectations formulated and stated by the patient" (Peplau, 1990, p. 96).
"When the patient has clearly formulated an expectation, then ask 'What happened instead?' " (Peplau, 1990, p. 96).

| 11. Get Mr. Morrison to determine if changes might be needed in his career expectations. | The nurse should "consider which factors . . . are amenable to control" and then discuss with the client what change in expectations might be possible (Peplau, 1990, p. 96). |

Implementing

Documentation indicates the following client behaviors:

1. Mr. Morrison met with the nurse for one hour on a weekly basis.
2. Mr. Morrison's anxiety was reduced to the level at which he could sing during performances.
3. Mr. Morrison recognizes the connection between his physiological symptoms and the feelings of anxiety.
4. Mr. Morrison recognizes that a change in his career expectations for the future may be needed, but that at the present time he should still be able to fulfill his singing engagements at a satisfactory level.

Documentation includes the following implementation of nursing actions:

1. The nurse met with Mr. Morrison each week at the appointed time with the exception of one week when there was a conflict in the scheduling.
2. The nursing actions were carried out essentially as planned during each session.

Evaluating

The client's progress will be evaluated by measuring the degree of anxiety reduction and by an increase in the client's ability to perform without experiencing incapacitating behaviors of anxiety. According to Belcher and Fish (1985) "although Peplau does not discuss evaluation per se, evaluation is an inherent factor in determining the status of readiness for the client to proceed through the resolution phase" (p. 86).

Product Evaluation (Extent that Goals and Predicted Outcomes were Met)

1. After 2 weeks of therapy Mr. Morrison reported a decrease in the diarrhea and feeling of choking.
2. After 2 weeks Mr. Morrison kept all his singing engagements and was able to perform without forgetting words of songs.

Process Evaluation

Nurse Focus (extent that planned nursing interventions and nursing actions were implemented).

1. The nurse was able to meet with the client each week; however, because of a conflict in staff scheduling, one appointment had to be changed. This was discussed with the client prior to the change and he was agreeable to the change.
2. The nurse was able to monitor personal anxiety and Mr. Morrison's anxiety during sessions with him.
3. The nurse was able to carry out nursing actions essentially as had been planned.

Client Focus (extent that etiology component of the nursing diagnosis statement was modified).

1. After one month he was able to verbalize connections between his perceptions of career failure and behaviors which caused him to feel anxious and to seek help.
2. He has indicated that he believes his singing performances will be satisfactory for a number of years to come. He also indicated that career expectations needed to be reconsidered, but he is still having difficulty accepting the idea that his ability to sing may one day diminish.

SUMMARY

This chapter has described the use of Peplau's theory in the care of an anxious client. Peplau encourages nurses to examine their own behaviors in interactions with their clients, thus promoting the nurse-patient relationship. She believes that this relationship is a therapeutic tool to be used to help clients reduce their anxiety. Peplau provides not only the theoretical aspects of anxiety but has developed nursing interventions that all nurses can learn to use with anxious clients.

REFERENCES

Belcher, J. R., & Fish, L. A. B. (1985). Hildegard E. Peplau. In J. B. George (Ed.) *Nursing theories: The base for professional nursing practice* (pp. 73–87). Englewood Cliffs, NJ: Prentice Hall.

Horney, K. (1937). *The neurotic personality of our time*. New York: W. W. Norton.

May, R. (1977). *The meaning of anxiety*. New York: W. W. Norton.

May, R., Angel, E., & Ellenberger, H. F. (Eds.). (1958). *Existence: A new dimension in psychiatry and psychology*. New York: Basic Books.

Murray, R. B., & Huelskoetter, M. M. (1991). *Psychiatric mental health nursing: Giving emotional care* (3rd ed.). Englewood Cliffs, NJ: Prentice Hall.

Peplau, H. E. (1952). *Interpersonal relations in nursing*. New York: G. P. Putnam & Sons.

Peplau, H. E. (1963). A working definition of anxiety. In S. F. Burd & M. A. Marshall (Eds.) *Some clinical approaches to psychiatric nursing* (pp. 323–327). New York: Macmillan.

Peplau, H. E. (1979). Manifestations of anxiety and intervention. In W. E. Field (Ed.) *The psychotherapy of Hildegard E. Peplau* (pp. 17–24). New Braunfels, TX: PSF Productions.[1]

Peplau, H. E. (1987). Interpersonal constructs for nursing practice. *Nurse Education Today*, 7, 201–208.

Peplau H. E. (1989a). Interpersonal relationships: The purpose and characteristics of professional nursing. In A. W. O'Toole & S. R. Welt (Eds.) *Interpersonal theory in nursing practice: Selected works of Hildegard E. Peplau* (pp. 42–55). New York: Springer Publishing Co.[2]

Peplau H. E. (1989b). Therapeutic nurse-patient interaction. In A. W. O'Toole & S. R. Welt (Eds.) *Interpersonal theory in nursing practice: Selected works of Hildegard E. Paplau* (pp. 192–204). New York: Springer Publishing Co.[3]

Peplau H. E. (1990). Interpersonal relations model: Principles and general applications. In W. Reynolds & D. Cormack (Eds.) *Psychiatric and mental health nursing: Theory and practice* (pp. 87–132). London: Chapman & Hall.

Sullivan, H. S. (1953). *The interpersonal theory of psychiatry*. New York: Norton.

Wilson, H. S., & Kneisl, C. R. (1989). *Psychiatric nursing*. Menlo Park, CA: Addison-Wesley.

Ziegler, S. M., Vaughan-Wrobel, B. C. & Erlen, J. S. (1986). *Nursing process, nursing diagnosis, and nursing knowledge: Avenues to autonomy*. Norwalk, CT: Appleton-Century-Crofts.

[1] Selected material from Hildegard Peplau's lectures.
[2] Adapted and edited version of a paper presented by Hildegard Peplau at the Council of Hospital Services, District of Columbia-Delaware Hospital Association, Washington D.C., February, 1965.
[3] Edited paper of Hildegard Peplau presented at the Hamilton Psychiatric Hospital, Hamilton, Ontario, April, 1984.

SUGGESTED READINGS

Horney, K. (1939). *New ways in psychoanalysis*. New York: W. W. Norton.
Horney, K. (1945). *Our inner conflicts.* New York: W. W. Norton.
May, R. (1969). *Love and will*. New York: W. W. Norton.
May, R. (1983). Anxiety and stress. In H. Selye (Ed.) *Selye's guide to stress research* (vol. 2). New York: Scientific and Academic Editions.

Chapter 9

Lewin's Field Theory with Emphasis on Change

Susan Goad and Lois Hough

In some instances a group of nurses working together will observe a need for change and work to initiate it of their own volition. In other instances an event in the environment impinges upon a group of nurses and change must occur even though it is not desired. Whether the impetus for change is voluntary or involuntary, the process through which people move to achieve change is the same.

The case of Bellwether General Hospital illustrates the management of a negative response of a group of nurses to the projected introduction of graduate and undergraduate nursing students into their environment. Several theories, which might be selected to guide the intervention, are considered. Lewin's Field Theory is applied to the Bellwether General Hospital case.

CASE SITUATION

Bellwether General Hospital opened 2 years ago. It is located in a growing community near a large metropolitan area. The medical, nursing, occupational therapy, and physical therapy schools of the state university are located in the nearby city. In their strategic plan the directors of Bellwether projected a liaison with the university to cooperate in the education of health professionals. Contract talks are in progress. While some minor details remain to be resolved, students from all four health disciplines are scheduled to begin clinical practice experiences starting in the fall semester 3 months hence.

Case management is in place on the obstetric, surgical, orthopedic, psychiatric, and all but one of the medical units. The nurses and physicians on these units worked diligently to develop and refine the critical pathways for their respective services. The system is working very well. The physicians are satisfied with the care their patients receive; the patients are responding well to their treatment. The nurses are pleased to be directing their energies toward a method of care they were influential in devising. Besides being a source of pride the case management system provides an opportunity for advancement. Case managers are selected from the staff on the basis of ability, without regard for educational preparation. The staff is divided about equally between associate and baccalaureate degree nurses. The work is satisfying and morale is high.

When word of the impending student affiliations circulates around the hospital, the various nursing units are not receptive to the idea. On the orthopedic unit there is overt hostility. The prospect of undergraduate student nurses is seen as disruptive, time-consuming, and a threat to the smoothness of the unit's operation. The prospect of graduate students on the unit is seen as a threat to staff nurses' hopes of becoming case managers in the future. With potentially better qualified nurses on site, the resident staff nurses anticipate they will be at a disadvantage when case manager positions become available.

The head nurse and clinical nurse specialist discuss what has occurred. They determine there is a need to plan a course of action that will introduce planned change to the nursing staff on the orthopedic unit.

PATTERNING CUES FROM CLIENT CASE

Before the Clinical Nurse Specialist (CNS) and Head Nurse (HN) can attempt to devise a plan for a receptive introduction of student nurses into the Orthopedic Unit, they must first determine why staff view the impending event as potentially disruptive. After the reason is identified, the CNS and HN can consider possible theories that will generate intervention strategies to apply to the situation in order to bring about a predictable and desired outcome.

The Orthopedic Unit is functioning well. The physicians and nurses have worked out mutually satisfactory systems and procedures. On a specific date in the near future outsiders will be introduced into this smoothly functioning setting. How this event will affect the unit's operation and its personnel is unknown. Therefore, staff are exhibiting a negative reaction to the imminent alteration of the status quo.

As a first step the CNS and HN identify cues from which to pattern the identity of the problem. Cues in this case consist of the following:

- Nurses have heavy investment in unit's processes
- Morale is high
- Nurses' work is satisfying
- Nurses have hope for advancement
- Introduction of graduate and undergraduate student nurses is inevitable
- Widespread dissatisfaction with prospect of students because of negative expectations
- Overt hostility on Orthopedic Unit
- Number of academically prepared nurses will increase
- Competition from better prepared nurses on site.

The assembly of cues into related clusters results in identifying a pattern of resistance to an impending change. Since the change is not precipitate, the CNS and HN can work with the staff to alter their perceptions of the impact of the change. With a change of perception about the event, there can be an expected change in behavior toward the event. The CNS and HN consider possible theories that could be applied to remedy the situation.

SELECTED RELEVANT THEORIES

The authors considered several theories to determine which one most nearly explains a current situation, provides direction for intervention, and predicts an expected outcome. Several theoretical frameworks are applicable to the clinical situation.

Von Bertalanffy's Systems Theory

Ludwig von Bertalanffy, a theoretical biologist, proposed general systems theory in 1950. He applied universal principles to the open system, regardless of the type of system, nature of the component elements, or the relationships among the elements. According to von Bertalanffy (1968), general systems theory serves as a model for viewing the interaction between man and his environment.

The hospital organization can be viewed as an open system. Modern organization theory conceptualizes the hospital organization as a complex social system that is a part of the suprasystem of society. Kast and Rosenzweig (1985) applied general systems theory to organizations. The organization is an integrated whole of mutually dependent parts that exchange information and energy with the environment. The constant input of new information from the environment results in inevitable change. A change in one part of the system affects the other subsystems. Therefore, management process can be considered as a series of interrelated elements that interact within the organizational environment.

Equilibrium occurs when the organization balances the forces operating on it and within its internal organization. The subsystems experience stress, produced in part by the opposing forces. The systems framework is useful for analyzing change needed in health care organizations.

The change agent must develop systems thinking and analyze the flow of information into the system. The change agent must understand that the whole is greater than the sum of its parts. The change agent analyzes variables affecting the system, which may be internal or environmental. Systems framework also directs the subsystems and hierarchical activities. Thus, the change agent assesses the suprasystem and transactions occurring at all levels of the system. For example, environmental variables such as the introduction of nursing students, affect the flow of the systems.

Systems theory provides a framework for viewing and interpreting the interactions among the subsystems of the organization. However, systems theory is an abstract theory and does not provide directions for interventions. Therefore, another theory, or combination of theories, must be utilized to generate interventions.

Lippitt's Planned Change

Another theoretical approach that may be applicable to the case situation is Gordon Lippitt's (1973) theory of planned change. According to Lippitt, planned change or "neomobilistic" change is defined as a conscious, planned effort which moves a system, an organization, or an individual in a new direction. Lippitt's theory may be used with an individual, group, or institution.

Lippitt's theory expands the work of Kurt Lewin's field theory. According to Lippitt, planned change is goal-directed. The change agent is a person skilled in the theory of planned change who initiates and accomplishes the change. The change agent uses a process of confrontation to accomplish the change. Confrontation is the change agent's involvement with people and situations, the initiation of the process, and action, not simply reaction. Those forces which originate inside the organization, system, or individual and which facilitate change, are termed driving forces. Restraining forces are those forces originating inside the organization or the environment that impede change.

There are seven phases in Lippitt's theory. The phases do not possess rigid boundaries, rather movement may flow back and forth between the phases. The first phase involves identification and diagnosis of the problem. All persons affected by the change should have an opportunity to help identify the problem. In phase two, the change agent assesses the client systems motivation and capacity for change. In phase three, the initiator of change assesses his or her ability to help in a situation. The change agent's motivation, experience, credentials, and personality are important factors in this assessment. The change agent selects progressive change objectives in phase four. The change agent then chooses an appropriate role in phase five. The change agent may be actively involved in the implementation of change, serve as an expert by gathering and providing data, or function as a liaison within the organization. Phase six involves maintenance of the change. The last (seventh) phase is termination of the helping relationship. The change agent withdraws from the situation, leaving the client system alone to maintain the change. Prior to the termination individuals with power are identified to maintain the change.

Because Lippitt's theory involves a helping relationship, it is more appropriate for a client or one-to-one relationship. The case situation involves several groups of nurses on the unit; therefore, a more global approach is indicated.

Lewin's Change Theory

Kurt Lewin, a German psychologist, worked at the Massachusetts Institute of Technology. His Field Theory was never fully drawn together in his life time. He died in 1947; his works were not translated and published until 1951. Field Theory, as developed by Lewin, is an attempt to unify the field of psychology in a precise and logical manner through the analysis of causal relations and the development of scientific constructs. The analysis of causal relations leads to an understanding of the dynamics of social situations. Since this chapter deals only with the social phenomenon of planned change, explanation of Lewin's Field Theory is limited to that portion commonly referred to as Change Theory. Change theory represents a special application of field theory to the process involved in altering an event or events experienced by a group in a social situation (Lewin, 1951a).

In organized situations or institutions events flow through defined social channels (Lewin, 1951a). Within the channels are natural gates that are either managed by gatekeepers or controlled by rules. Both gatekeepers and rules are subject to boundary conditions. These boundaries determine the extent of power the gatekeepers/rules can exercise in determining who or what may pass through the gates. The amount of power can be altered by influencing or replacing the gatekeepers or changing the rules. However, if neither option is viable, then situation altering social circumstances are permitted to pass through the gates. The prevailing condition(s) or status quo may be forced to experience unplanned, or preferably planned, change.

Central to change theory is the concept of the force field (Lewin, 1951b). Force field is a present social situation with all its properties existing over a period of time. These properties represent two levels of forces having current impact. Past, present, and future events represent the reality forces level. Hopes, aspirations and emotional investments represent the irreality level of forces.

Lewin (1951a) referred to these two levels of forces as quasi-stationary forces. These forces have both direction and velocity. The resultants of quasi-stationary forces become the quasi-stationary processes that determine whether or not a particular event occurring in a social context is in a state of stability. The state of stability generated by the quasi-stationary processes is called quasi-stationary equilibrium. The quasi-stationary process which moves toward intensifying a particular event is composed of the quasi-stationary forces Lewin termed driving forces; the quasi-stationary forces combining to diminish the intensity of an event he called restraining forces. The occurrence of a quasi-stationary equilibrium is dependent upon whether or not the resultants of the restraining and driving forces are equal.

The use of "quasi-stationary" reflects Lewin's perception that social situations do not remain static and that without intervention, they will experience evolutionary change over time. However, when the quasi-stationary equilibrium is undesirable, the change process can be expedited using Lewin's (1951c) approach to analysis of the social field.

With time and usage the terminology coined by Lewin and translated by Cartwright has evolved to simpler expressions. The quasi-stationary forces are referred to as driving and restraining forces. The quasi-stationary equilibrium is referred to as the status quo. The social situation containing the quasi-stationary forces and quasi-stationary equilibrium is the force field. The social channels with gates are the various events, controlled by people or rules, operating on a force field. The more contemporary terms are used in describing the dynamics of Lewin's Change Theory.

Planned change results from a carefully planned, logical effort by one or more persons deliberately to alter a situation (Lewin, 1951d). The term change agent, though not coined by Lewin, has come to mean a responsible person who moves those to be affected by the change through the stages of change in a logical manner. Initiation and execution of the change process should satisfy the following rules:

1. There should be a good reason for implementing change.
2. Change should be a gradual process.
3. Individuals who may be affected by the change should be involved in planning for it.

DESCRIPTION OF LEWIN'S CHANGE THEORY

Major Concepts

The selected concepts of Lewin's Change Theory are organized under the major concepts of force field, motivators, stages, and change agent. Table 9.1 presents a summary of the selected major concepts with their associated

Table 9.1   Selected Concepts of Lewin's Change Theory

Force Field
   Driving Forces
   Restraining Forces
   Status quo
Motivators
   Confirmation of non-accomplishment
   Confirmation of lack of obtainment
   Confirmation of lack of growth or maturation
Stages
   Unfreezing
   Moving
   Refreezing
Change Agent

subconcepts. Lewin's Field Theory is a highly complex and encompassing theory. This chapter will only deal with the part concerned with change.

Theoretical Definition of Major Concepts

Definitions are provided for the major concepts and subconcepts.

Force Field

The Force Field consists of all the behavior of a group in its environment during a given period of time. The effect of this interaction is explained by the concepts driving forces, restraining forces, and status quo.

1. *Driving forces* are the past, present, and future elements along with hopes, aspirations, and emotional investments which tend to effect a social event in a positive direction.
2. *Restraining forces* are the past, present, and future elements along with hopes, aspirations, and emotional investments which tend to effect a social event in a negative direction.
3. *Status quo* is a dynamic equilibrium composed of a balance between the driving and restraining forces.

Lewin (1951d) asserted that the forces prevent revolutionary change and in fact permit equilibrium or status quo in the system.

Motivators

Motivators are the initial stimuli which convince the concerned parties there is a need for change. There are three categories of motivators:

1. *Confirmation of non-accomplishment*—information which confirms the fact that the desired job is not being accomplished.
2. *Confirmation of lack of obtainment*—information that confirms the fact that what is wanted, needed, or expected, is not obtained.

3. *Confirmation of lack of growth or motivation*—information that confirms the fact that growth or maturation is not being achieved.

Stages

According to Lewin (1951d), planned change occurs in three stages. These are termed unfreezing, moving, and refreezing. (Freezing is now commonly referred to as refreezing.) These three stages must occur before the planned change becomes a part of the system.

1. *Unfreezing*. The stage in the change process during which the change agents create dissatisfaction followed by inspiring the motivation to accept some type of change. The three basic motivators that initiate unfreezing demonstrate that either the status quo does not provide what is wanted, needed, or expected; does not achieve task accomplishment; or does not promote growth or maturation. This unfreezing step represents a necessary step in stimulating people to recognize the need for change.

2. *Moving*. The second step of change theory is a cognitive redefinition by the participants of attitude and behavior toward the planned change. Individuals have what Lewin (1951d) refers to as habits of social action and thinking. These are the source of inner resistance to change. In order to overcome this resistance, it is necessary to change the values of the group of which the individual is a member. This is best accomplished by involvement of the group in the change process or encouraging group decision making.

3. *Refreezing* (Freezing). This is the stage during which the new behaviors are practiced and reinforced. New behavior patterns are integrated into the participants. This is the final link in the three-stage related process. What began with dissatisfaction evolved into motivation, leading to alteration of values, followed by alteration of behavior. The decision to stick to self-generated decisions also helps the new behavior persist.

Change Agent

Change agent is an individual who is skilled in change theory and the practice of planned change. This title is not a component of change theory, but is inferred from the theory. From an analysis of the force field, the change agent identifies the problem and institutes planned change by examining the driving and restraining forces that maintain the problem situation.

Examples of Concepts Relevant to Role Practice

Four major concepts of the theory are illustrated in the following examples. The examples are representative of a variety of nursing settings.

Force Field

A head nurse of an oncology unit is the manager of all the personnel and patients in a designated time frame (force field). Some dynamics occurring on the unit are coalitions that have developed among the unit's personnel over time, emergence of an informal leader, expectations of promotion or pay raise (driving forces), personal and group animosity, and personnel cutbacks (restraining forces). These result in a condition of stability with nurses delivering quality care with minimal tardiness and absenteeism (status quo).

Motivators

The physicians have indicated they are receptive to the nurses administering inpatient chemotherapy. The head nurse calls a meeting and presents the idea to the staff. In order for the staff to be receptive to the idea, she utilizes motivators. She accomplishes this using the following information: they are unable to perform the chemotherapy now (confirmation of non-accomplishment); some nurses are not certified in this hospital to administer chemotherapy (confirmation of lack of obtainment); certification in chemotherapy is routine for oncology nurses (confirmation of lack of growth).

Stages

However, preliminary to the nurses administering chemotherapy is their certification in chemotherapy (unfreezing). At the meeting the head nurse and staff generate and evaluate alternatives and develop a plan for obtaining the necessary certification (moving). Following completion of necessary course work, the Clinical Nurse Specialist (change agent) acts as a support person and reinforces knowledge from the certification program. The nurses who demonstrate competency in chemotherapy receive a pay raise (refreezing).

Change Agent

The head nurse, in initiating and directing the effort to obtain certification for administration of chemotherapy, has acted as a change agent. She accomplished the change process beginning with analysis of the force field, application of motivators, and providing direction through the stages of the change process.

Major Relational Statements

This section identifies the major relational statements of Lewin's change theory.

1. To alter the status quo, the dynamic equilibrium developed by the balance between driving and restraining forces must be altered.
2. If the group value(s) is changed, the individual members of the group are more likely to accept the change than if change is offered to individuals alone.
3. It is preferable to diminish the strength of the restraining forces rather than increase the strength of the driving forces in order to achieve change (Lewin, in Cartwright, 1951).
4. For planned change to occur, the three stages of unfreezing, moving, and refreezing must be enacted.
5. The need for change must be recognized by the people involved in the change before the planned change process can be initiated.
6. To develop a status quo, elements of past, current, and future components must be in oppositional equilibrium.
7. If new behavior is to become stable, it must be reinforced by means of positive feedback, encouragement, or constructive criticism.

IMPLICATIONS OF LEWIN'S CHANGE THEORY
FOR ROLE PRACTICE

Change theory is a useful theory for the practice of nursing roles in clinical settings. As a theory useful for practice, it is compatible with the problem-solving process of assessing, problem defining, planning, implementing, and evaluating. These steps parallel the steps of the nursing process, differing only by the exchange of problem defining for nursing diagnosis.

Factors to be Assessed and Methods of Assessing

The first factor to be assessed is to determine whether or not a particular status quo is in need of change. If the answer is yes, then the change agent needs to identify the nature and relative strength of the driving and restraining forces operating in the force field. From the analysis a determination is made of which one or several restraining forces is to be altered in order for the desired change to occur (Lewin, 1951d).

Methods of assessment include observations, interviews, or record review. Any methods, which elicit information about reality and irreality impinging on the status quo, could be used. This data will eventually be arranged on a force field chart.

A force field chart consists of a central line which represents the status quo. There are five lines above and below the central status quo line. Each line represents a degree of intensity of a force impinging on the status quo. The lines are numbered 1 to 5, with the first lines above and below the central line assigned the value of "1". The second lines above and below are assigned the value of "2," and so on until the fifth set of lines is numbered. The set of lines above center (status quo) are used to chart restraining forces, and those below center are used to chart the driving forces.

The strength of both the restraining and driving forces is determined from the same decision rule in order to assign consistent values to the strength of the restraining and driving forces (Lewin, 1951d). To accomplish this, a scale should be developed. The scale describes a continuum of weakness to strength using terms applicable to the given situation. The change agents would devise something similar to the following:

1. Very little influence on change.
2. Some influence on change.

3. Moderate influence on change.
4. Important influence on change.
5. Major influence on change.

An arrow originating from the assigned value and terminating at the central line is placed on the chart above or below the central line, depending on whether it represents a driving or restraining force.

Theory-Specific Problem Definition

From these data, the change agents define the specific problem. The problem represents a difference between the current status quo and the desired status quo (La Monica, 1990).

Change theory directs problem defining to start with the development of a force field analysis. All those factors having a direct bearing on the problem are identified. From these three sources—the problem itself, the related personnel, and the associated factors—the target of change is selected.

Problem Resolution Plan

The third step in the problem-solving approach utilized by the change agent is planning. The target of change is selected (restraining force) from the force field analysis and the appropriate motivator is chosen to initiate the change process. The change agent devises interventions which activate motivation. When signs of unfreezing emerge, the interventions to facilitate moving are applied. Finally, reinforcers are selected to encourage continuation of the desired change.

Implementation of the Plan

The next step in the problem-solving process is implementing or executing the planned interventions. To initiate unfreezing, the change agents apply one of the basic motivators. These steps are described in Table 9.2. According to Lewin (1951d), a successful change involves three steps: unfreezing

Table 9.2 The Steps of Change Theory and Relevant Interventions

Steps	Relevant Interventions
Unfreezing	Identify the need for change. Apply specific motivators to convince and develop desire to change.
Moving	Assess environment. Plan strategies. Facilitate interventions.
Refreezing	Learned behaviors reinforced.

the present level, moving to the new level, and refreezing group life on the new level.

Evaluation of the Plan

The final step in the problem-solving process is evaluating. Evaluation may be either outcome evaluation or process evaluation, or both. Outcome evaluation is the determination of whether or not there has been a change in behavior resulting in attainment of the new and desired status quo. Process evaluation is the determination of the adequacy of the change process intervention strategies applied.

THEORY DIRECTED ROLE PRACTICE IN THE BELLWETHER HOSPITAL CASE

The five steps of the problem-solving process and the steps of the change process according to Lewin are combined to resolve the problem presented in the Bellwether Hospital case. This combination of theory and the problem-solving process demonstrates an orderly and theoretical resolution of a problem.

Assessing

In the present situation, the change agents identified the driving and restraining forces with their respective weights and arrayed them on a force field. These are illustrated in Table 9.3 and Figure 9.1. (Not all forces from the

Table 9.3   Operative Forces in Force Field

Driving forces		WT		Restraining forces	WT
A.	High morale	3	A.	Addition of nursing students	5
B.	Investment in unit's operation	3	B.	Expectation of disruption to unit work flow	4
C.	Work satisfying	5	C.	Increased competition for case manager positions from better qualified nurses	3
D.	Hope of advancement	4	D.	Overtly hostile	3
Total		15			15

case are used.) Table 9.3. demonstrates three points. First, the most significant forces from the case are identified and placed into columns depending on whether they are viewed as driving or restraining forces. Second, using a decision rule, the strength of all the forces is estimated. Finally, the combined strengths of the driving and restraining forces are totaled. The value of 15 is obtained for both driving and restraining forces. This represents a stable status quo which will persist until planned change is initiated.

Figure 9.1. is a graphic representation of the information found in Table 9.3. The capitalized letters on the lines identify both driving and restraining forces. The length of the arrows corresponds to the respective strengths of the driving and restraining forces impinging on the status quo. This visualization of the force field is helpful in comprehending the totality of a given situation and targeting problem areas for intervention.

Problem Defining

The final part of the force field analysis is selecting the force to which to apply the change strategy. This is accomplished by selecting one or several forces from the restraining forces as suggested by Lewin (1951d). The restraining force chosen as the problem was the addition of nursing students on the unit. This restraining force was chosen because it was judged to have the greatest negative impact on the situation.

According to La Monica (1990) a problem is defined as the difference between what is actually happening in a situation and the optimal condition for the situation. The problem for the Bellwether case is as follows:

Actual: A well-running unit.

Optimal: Unit will continue to run well with the addition of nursing students.

Problem: Present staff are not prepared for the planned change, introduction of nursing students.

Goal: Staff prepared to incorporate students into the functioning of the unit.

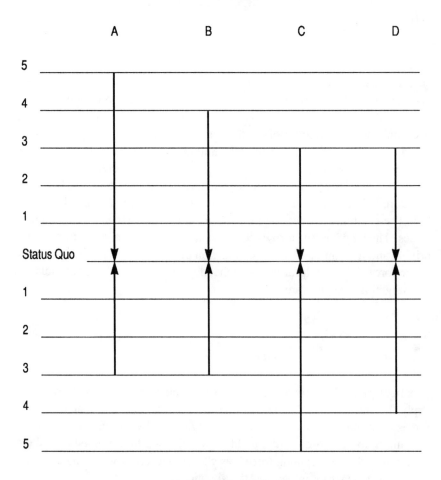

Figure 9.1 Force field analysis.

Currently the nursing staff is functioning in a case management mode. All personnel have contributed to the system and have a potential for advancement to case manager positions. The introduction of students is seen as threatening to the smoothness of the units' operation. The baccalaureate students' unfamiliarity with both nursing and with following the units' critical pathways for patient care is seen at the heart of the problem.

The gatekeeping function which determined that students would affiliate with Bellwether Hospital was at a level of administration to which the change agents have no access. However, preparing for implementing the change was within the purview of their role. The two lesser restraining forces are not included for intervention because of the likelihood that they will lose their impact when an acceptable planned change has occurred.

Planning

The change agents next devised a plan which would incorporate motivation to change and the steps of change theory (unfreezing, moving, refreezing) directed toward the targeted restraining force, addition of students. Also, the change agents derived a goal statement from the targeted restraining force. The goal statement is as follows: The staff will be prepared to incorporate students into the functioning of the unit.

The change agents begin by reviewing the three categories of motivators used to initiate the unfreezing step. Lewin (1951d) asserts that unfreezing of the present level may involve quite different problems in different situations. Demonstrating that the status quo is undesirable is not chosen because pointing out the staff's negative feelings about the potential disruption to the unit's work flow could make them defensive and heighten emotionalism on the unit. Absence of task achievement is not chosen because it cannot honestly be applied to the case situation. The remaining class of motivators, inadequate growth and maturation, does have relevance to the case situation.

The change agents develop a plan based on three points to stimulate interest in the impending arrival of undergraduate and graduate nursing students. The points are:

1. Professionals have an obligation to contribute to the education of succeeding generations of students.
2. Students are stimulating and their presence challenges staff to be current and to grow.

3. Patients can benefit from enhanced nursing care, if students are methodically incorporated into the case management team.

To make the staff aware of these points, the change agents discuss them informally whenever an opportunity presents itself. The staff is provided with literature that supports one or more of the points to be made. Finally, an in-service program is presented to the staff by an educator from the university, who describes how nursing students can be utilized in case management teams. The educator's presentation is taped and available for showing to all personnel not present at the live presentation. When the staff shows signs of interest in the incoming students, the unfreezing stage is accomplished.

The change agents set up a series of meetings utilizing group process strategies so that all staff members can contribute to developing a plan for methodically incorporating the two levels of students into the unit's case management team. Lewin (1951d) holds that dealing with groups facilitates change more readily than dealing with individuals. During continuing meetings the following plan evolves:

1. The role for undergraduate nursing students will be as team members.
2. The role for graduate students will be as case managers.
3. The staff will serve as mentors to both levels of students.
4. A standardized orientation schedule will be developed.
5. A committee will be organized to develop the orientation schedule.
6. The CNS will present sessions to the staff to teach them the art of mentoring.

The involvement of the staff in preparing for the incoming students constitutes the moving step of the change process.

Implementing

The fall semester begins and only undergraduate students arrive on the unit. The orientation schedule is operationalized. At its inception there is confusion because the original plan did not include the role of university faculty assigned with the students. An emergency meeting is held between the change agents and faculty members to resolve the differences in expectations. After reviewing the orientation schedule, the faculty members conceded the orientation role to the CNS and staff. Mentors were assigned by the Head Nurse. As staff members worked cooperatively with the students, the change agents praised their exemplary behaviors as reinforcers. In general the presence of students did not disrupt unit work flow. At the end of the semester the student and mentor pairs parted reluctantly. The staff looked forward to the next group of incoming students. This perception of the impact of the students on unit work flow represents the third step, refreezing, of the change process.

The course of action taken to implement planned change, introducing students into a smoothly running unit, did not alter unit work flow. The planned change process of initiation of unfreezing through exposure to a motivator, movement toward change through participation, and accomplishment of change by stabilizing refreezing through the utilization of reinforcements demonstrates application of Lewin's field theory.

Evaluating

The final step in the problem-solving process is determining if the goal has been achieved and how well the interventions used contributed to achieving the goal. This is accomplished through outcome and process evaluation. Outcome evaluation is the determination of whether or not there has been a change in behavior resulting in attainment of the new and desired status quo. The original goal was that the staff would be prepared to incorporate students into the functioning of the unit. Evidence that the goal was achieved was that the introduction of students occurred without incident. Further, the change agents observed cohesiveness and harmony in the student–mentor pairs.

Process evaluation is the determination of the adequacy of the intervention strategies. In this situation, group process and teaching strategies were used to bring about change. The group process strategy was evaluated in terms of the adequacy of the orientation schedule that was produced. There was insufficient expertise in the group because of the omission of provision for the role of the university-based clinical instructor. The teaching strategy— preparation for mentorship—was evaluated at the end of the presentations by using a formal feedback sheet. At the end of the semester it was informally noted that the mentored-pairs had performed successfully.

SUMMARY

This chapter has described change theory and demonstrated its application to a nursing related situation. In this case the introduction of nursing students represented a case of involuntary change to a unit's staff. It matters not whether nurses are faced with mandated or self-generated change, Lewin's theory is useful to apply to any impending change in a health care setting.

REFERENCES

Cartwright, D. (1951). Forward. In D. Cartwright (Ed.) *Field theory in social science: Selected theoretical papers by Kurt Lewin,* (pp. vii–xv). New York: Harper & Brothers.[1]

Kast, F. F., & Rosenzweig, J. E. (1985). *Organization and management.* New York: McGraw-Hill.

La Monica, E. (1990). *Management in nursing.* New York: Springer Publishing Co.

Lewin, K. (1951a). Psychological ecology. In D. Cartwright (Ed.) *Field theory in social science: Selected theoretical papers by Kurt Lewin.* (pp. 170–187). New York: Harper & Brothers.

Lewin K. (1951b). Behavior and development as a function of the total situation. In D. Cartwright (Ed.) *Field theory in social science: Selected theoretical papers by Kurt Lewin.* (pp. 238–304). New York: Harper & Brothers.

Lewin, K. (1951c). Defining the field at a given time. In D. Cartwright (Ed.) *Field theory in social science: Selected theoretical papers by Kurt Lewin.* (pp. 43–59). New York: Harper & Brothers.

Lewin, K. (1951d). Frontiers in group dynamics. In D. Cartwright (Ed.) *Field theory in social science: Selected theoretical papers by Kurt Lewin.* (pp. 188–237). New York: Harper & Brothers.

Lippitt, G. L. (1973). *Visualizing change.* La Jolla, CA: University Associates.

von Bertalanffy, L. (1968). *General systems theory.* New York: Braziller.

This book is a collection of papers that Kurt Lewin published in various sources. Most of the papers cited in this chapter were originally published in the 1940s.

SUGGESTED READINGS

Gruce, J. (1987). A systems look at infection control. *Nursing Management, 18*(3), 50–51.

Kast, F. E., & Rosenzweig, J. E. (1981). General systems theory: Applications for organization and management. *Journal of Nursing Administration, 11*(7), 32–41.

McClure, M. L. (1984). Managing the professional nurse, Part I. *Journal of Nursing Administration, 14*(2), 15–20.

McClure, M. L. (1984). Managing the professional nurse, Part II. *Journal of Nursing Administration, 14*(3), 11–25.

Putt, A. M. (1978). *General systems theory: A guide for nursing.* Boston: Little, Brown, and Company.

Welch, L. B. (1979). Planned change in nursing: The theory. *Nursing clinics of North America, 14*(2), 307–321.

CHAPTER 10

Thomas' Conflict Theory

Lois Hough and Susan Goad

Whenever human beings come together, either as individuals or in groups, conflict may arise. The conflict occurs because each of the parties is following a personal agenda. Success or failure in the pursuit of one party's agenda can create a hazard to the other's pursuit of an agenda. How the parties handle conflict determines whether or not the occurrence will have a constructive or destructive outcome.

The possibility of a constructive outcome demonstrates that not all conflict is undesirable. At a controlled level conflict can be interesting, even stimulating. Diverse opinions are aired, ideas challenged, and mental capacity exercised. In decision-making situations the resolution of conflicting positions often contributes to more creative solutions. With uncontrolled levels of conflict, however, aggressive behavior may emerge with possibly destructive results. In situations that have escalated to an aggressive level, a definitive intervention becomes imperative.

The size, impersonality, and intensity within a modern day hospital generates many situations which may evolve into conflict situations between nurses or nurses and other members of a hospital staff. An efficient approach to conflict resolution is the application of a conflict theory based directed intervention. This chapter provides an overview of the conflict theories of Pondy (1967), Filley (1975) and Thomas (1976). The conflict theory of Thomas is used to demonstrate in detail the conflict resolution in a case.

199

CASE SITUATION

Fogram General Hospital (FGH) was established in 1928 as a 350-bed hospital. It is located in a medium-sized town surrounded by a prosperous rural area. FGH served the more conservative and affluent members of this community. Medical and obstetric services were provided and minor and non-heroic major surgery was performed. There were no intensive care units. If a medical or a surgical patient required close supervision, the recovery room doubled as an intensive care service. The hospital maintained no emergency department. In general the hospital was well-staffed and the atmosphere seldom stressful.

Some of the routines evolved over the years included night shift responsibility for patient care and the following tasks:

1. 6:00 A.M. temperatures
2. 24-hour summation of intakes and outputs
3. diet requests for breakfast meal, NPO's, specials, and generals
4. 24-hour summation of staff attendance
5. 24-hour summation of bed occupancy
6. 24-hour count of supply consumption
7. 24-hour count of narcotic and stock medications consumption
8. 24-hour count of specimen container consumption
9. 24-hour status report of regular and special equipment on the unit
10. Inventory of linens remaining in the cupboard
11. Inventory of supplies remaining on the supply shelves.

On the basis of these reports and inventories, units were restocked, billings posted, personnel benefits credited, and patient services rendered. These many activities performed by the night nurses were the keystone to the functioning of departments throughout FGH.

FGH was purchased by Kutani Megaconglomerate Incorporated. During the past 2 years the following changes have occurred:

1. The large salon areas on both wings on each of three floors were remodeled to add ten beds each, increasing overall hospital bed capacity by 60.
2. The salon area on the first floor was converted to an emergency department.
3. One salon area on the second floor was used for enlargement of the operating suite and recovery room. The other was remodeled into a

surgical intensive care unit and a combined medical and coronary care intensive care unit.

The hospital administrator has recruited younger and more aggressive surgeons to FGH's staff. The new ICUs are transferring a steady stream of acutely ill patients to the units. The emergency department also admits acutely ill and severely traumatized patients to the units.

While the numbers and kinds of patients at FGH have changed, the prevailing conditions have not. A few new nurses were added to staff the OR, ICUs and ER. Essentially, no additional staff was hired for the remodeled units now populated with more and sicker patients. Also, there was no provision for the staff to upgrade their nursing skills to meet new job demands. The paperwork routines have remained unchanged while the hospital organization has undergone drastic change. As a result the following situation has developed.

The night nurses cannot give care to more and sicker patients and complete all the summaries and inventories expected of them. This results in incomplete charting, late or omitted reports to other departments, and disruption of the routines in the various supply services. The system failure has generated conflict within nursing units and between nursing units and other hospital departments.

There are arguments, finger-pointing, and petty acts of spite. Personnel feel frustrated. In such an unpleasant environment morale is low. The Director of Nursing (DON) has tried repeatedly to impress the Hospital administrator with the gravity and urgency of the situation. The DON points out that incident reports are increasing in number and that the overloaded nurses are making more mistakes. An attitude of "it's only a matter of time until something dreadful happens" is prevalent. The administrator finally perceives the seriousness of the situation and agrees to request a nurse consultant from corporate headquarters.

PATTERNING CUES FROM CASE SITUATION

Fogram General Hospital (FGH) has been dragged kicking and screaming into the twentieth century. The acuity level of the patient mix is markedly increased. The number of nursing personnel has not increased nor has their skill level. The rules and procedures within which the hospital personnel function are the result of evolutionary change over the last 60 to 70 years.

The evolutionary change process is unable to produce rule and procedure changes apace with the revolutionary change that has occurred in FGH.

The deficit in procedural change results in a chain reaction of failures. The night nurses are pressured by hospital routines and personal professional standards to accomplish all the tasks in the present that they had accomplished in the past. This cannot occur because more of their time is spent at patients' bedsides. The night nurses do as much as they can and report to the day shift. There are exchanges of unpleasantness as the day shift feels they are making up for neglectful night nurses. The unpleasantness is repeated throughout the day as tardy or nonexistent reports create frustration in departments other than nursing.

As the personnel in all departments try to do their jobs, they perceive others creating obstacles. These obstacles hinder performance and may be perceived as a threat to personal status, even job security. A defensive or aggressive posture is assumed. Where threatening conditions prevail, the worst in people emerges. In their exchanges, the parties in conflict are not using behaviors that will lead to conflict resolution. All parties—nurses and other hospital personnel—are faced with a situation generating pressures and constraints which block their style of problem solving. A nurse consultant is called in to diagnose the situation and recommend resolution strategies.

SELECTED RELEVANT THEORIES

Several theories are explored for resolution of the problem in the case situation. These are described, with an in-depth explanation of Thomas' conflict theory, the theory chosen by the authors as most applicable to the case situation.

Pondy's General Theory of Conflict

Pondy (1967) developed a general theory of conflict in the context of three conceptual models: a bargaining model, referring to parties in an interest-group relationship that are in competition for resources; the bureaucratic model, which is applicable to parties in a superior-subordinate relationship; and a systems model dealing with parties in a lateral or working relationship.

Pondy defines conflict as a dynamic process that consists of a series of episodes between two or more individuals. Each episode begins with conditions that have conflict potentials. The individuals in the relationship may not know the basis of the conflict, and may not develop hostile feelings for one another. Their behavior may exhibit a variety of conflicting traits. Each episode leaves an aftermath which will affect succeeding episodes. Therefore, each conflict episode includes stages of latency, feeling perception, manifestation, and aftermath. Each of these stages will now be explained.

Three basic types of latent conflict exist in organizations: competition for scarce resources; drives for autonomy; and divergence of subunit goals when two parties who must cooperate on some joint project are unable to reach consensus. Pondy (1967) also asserts that another form of latent conflict is role conflict. Perceived conflict may exist when no conditions of latent conflict exist. Perceived conflict is said to exist from the parties misunderstanding of each others' true position. Conflict becomes felt or personalized when the whole personality of the individual is involved in the relationship.

Manifest conflict consists of behavior, such as open aggression, which frustrates the goals of some of the other participants. The end of the conflict episode, or aftermath, may consist of laying the behavior for a more cooperative relationship. On the other hand, the aftermath may aggravate relations and explode into a more serious situation.

Conflict resolution techniques depend on the nature of the conflict. Organization members may withdraw from the organization, altering existing relationships, or they may change values in the context of the existing relationships.

The Pondy theory focuses on organization conflict. Pondy defines conflict as a dynamic process during which the parties involved may or may not be aware of the source of the problem causing dissension between them. Resolution is dependent upon the alteration of relationships in the organization.

A nurse using Pondy's General Theory of Conflict would approach conflict resolution from the systems model, which deals with parties in working relationships. The nurse's intervention would focus on altering the relationship between the night nurses and other hospital departments. This would most likely take the form of removing or diminishing the dependency of the other hospital departments on the performance of articulating functions by the night nurses.

Filley's Interpersonal Conflict Resolution Theory

Filley (1975), drawing from the work of Corwin (1969) and Pondy (1967), developed his theory and incorporated an interpersonal conflict resolution model. Filley defined conflict as a process which takes place between two or more parties. Parties refers to individuals, groups, or organizations. If the gain of one party's goal is at the cost of the other party, or if the parties have different goals, then the resulting interaction between the parties could result in conflict.

Filley described various kinds of conflict. In a competitive conflict, only one party can achieve victory at the cost of the opponent's total loss. This situation is governed by a set of rules. On the other hand, a disruptive conflict does not follow a set of rules and the goal is not a win for one party. Instead, one party is intent on defeating or driving away the opponent. Filley depicted the following as the six steps in the conflict process:

1. Antecedent conditions are conditions that lead directly to or create opportunities for conflict to arise. These conditions, however, may also be present in the absence of conflict. Characteristics of social relationships that are antecedent conditions include conflict of inter-est, communication barriers, dependence of one party on the other, and unresolved prior conflicts.
2. Perceived conflict is the logical, impersonal, and objectively recognized set of conditions that exist within self or between parties that can cause conflict.
3. Felt conflict is the set of subjective feelings related to the conflict relationship.
4. The resulting action is manifest behavior in the form of aggression, nonassertion, competition, or debate.
5. Suppression or conflict resolution brings the conflict to an end.
6. Resolution aftermath encompasses the consequences of the conflict such as feelings, beliefs, and awards.

Filley described methods of conflict resolution and problem solving. Filley defined conflict resolution as the termination of manifest conflict between individual parties or groups. Problem-solving methods of conflict resolution are those which find ways to overcome obstacles in a high-quality decision-making manner. These decisions are acceptable to the parties involved in the conflict.

Three basic strategies are discussed for dealing with conflict: win–lose strategy, the lose–lose strategy, and the win–win strategy. The typical win–lose method is the exercise of authority. Another win–lose method is majority rule. In the lose–lose method neither side accomplishes what it wants, as each side only gets part of what it wants. The most popular lose–lose method is compromise, used as a negative term in Filley's model.

In contrast, win–win problem–solving strategies focus on goals. There are two forms of these strategies—consensus method and integrative decision-making methods. Consensus method occurs when a final solution is reached which is not unacceptable to anyone. Integrative decision method differs in degree rather than in kind from consensus method. Whereas consensus is utilized to solve judgmental problems, integrative method is used to sequence the decision process through a series of steps. The emphasis is on open and continual effort toward the objective and the need to resolve a conflict.

In essence Filley describes conflict as the result of parties perceiving interference with goal attainment. To overcome this interference, Filley recommends a problem-solving approach utilizing the specific interventions of consensus and integrative decision-making methods.

Applying Filley's Interpersonal Conflict Resolution Model to the FGH case, the nurse would involve representatives of the night nurses and affected departments to participate in joint problem-solving sessions. To achieve the most desirable form of conflict resolution, win–win, the nurse would foster incremental decision making to work through the complex of problems producing conflict.

Thomas' Conflict Theory

Originally the approach to dealing with conflict was situation specific. Each scientist studied one particular type of conflict such as a race riot, war, or intra-organizational disharmony. From such studies a fragmented, negatively oriented picture of conflict existed in the literature. Thomas (1976) reviewed the conflict literature and noted that many commonalties existed in what was thought to be a disparate body of information. From these commonalties Thomas synthesized a combined theoretical explanation of conflict and conflict management.

Thomas' intent was to generate an explanation of the conflict phenomenon and identify effective corrective measures. However, before he set about presenting the body of his work, Thomas acquainted the reader with an overview of the entire theory. It is necessary to have an idea of the whole in order to select the appropriate model with which to work. Additionally, the definitions related to conflict terminology have various meanings, so it is necessary to know Thomas' usage to interpret the theory correctly. Before presenting the particulars of the theory, a brief explanation and overview is presented.

Thomas (1976) specifically intends conflict to mean "the process which begins when one party perceives that the other has frustrated or is about to frustrate some concern of his" (p. 893). These concerns are referred to as issues and consist of, "disagreements, denial of a request, violation of an agreement, insult, active interference with performance, vying for scarce resources, breaking a norm, diminishing one's feeling, et cetera" (Thomas, 1976, p. 895).

Party means a social unit, which may consist of individuals, groups, or organizations. For the purpose of explaining the theory, Thomas uses the terms "conflict dyad" or"party and other" interchangeably. To frustrate means the placement of some form of impediment in the path of goal-seeking/attainment. The outcome of a conflict situation may be either constructive or destructive. Thomas generated the notion of dual outcome from his global view of the conflict literature. Prior to this, conflict was viewed only as a negative and destructive force.

Two models, a process model and a structural model, coexist within Thomas' theory to explain the whole of the conflict process. Inherent in both models is provision for the management of conflict.

In the process model the conflict process begins as an episode. A conflict episode is not an isolated event. Rather, it is several consecutive episodes that encompass a standardized chain of repetitive events. These episodes are interactive, since one party's behavior acts as the stimulus for the other to respond. The outcome of one set of episodes may impact on the outcomes of future conflict episodes.

The structural model differs from the process model mainly in that it is concerned with the underlying parameters of conflict episodes rather than the episodes themselves. At the center of the model, party and other are acting out conflict behavior. Four variables from the environment impinge on both party and other and influence the course of the conflict.

The Thomas Conflict Theory, with its dual descriptive models, encompasses the whole of the conflict phenomenon. Specific conflict situations come under the purview of either the process or structure model. For the purposes of this demonstration the focus of the resolution of the Fogram Hospital case will utilize only the process conflict model.

DESCRIPTION OF THOMAS' CONFLICT THEORY

Thomas used a pragmatic rather than an esoteric approach to describing his theory. The descriptions of concepts and subconcepts contain greater emphasis on operationalization than conceptualization. The reader finds that as both the main concepts and explanatory subconcepts are presented, Thomas provides a term by which like concepts and subconcepts can be recognized. For example, concepts, that describe an episode of conflict are referred to as events and are links in a chain of events. To make the reader more familiar with Thomas' work, these terms will be used and set off by quotation marks in the definitions of the conflict theory concepts and subconcepts.

Major Concepts

The process model of conflict depicts five major concepts which occur as a chain of events within a conflict episode from the view of one of the parties: frustration, conceptualization, behavior, other's reaction, and outcome. Conflict per se, the conflict dyad, and third party intervention are also defined in this section (Table 10.1).

Table 10.1   Selected concepts of Thomas' Conflict Theory

Conflict
Conflict dyad
Conflict episode
  Frustration
  Conceptualization
    Defining the issue
    Salient alternatives
  Behavior
    Orientation/desired result
      accommodative/appeasement
      avoidant/neglect
      collaborative/integration
      competitive/domination
      sharing/compromise
    Strategic objective
  Other's reaction
    Escalation/de-escalation
    Conflict management
  Outcome
    Conflict aftermath
    Long-term effects
Third party intervention
  Coloration
  De-escalation
  Confrontation

Theoretical Definitions of Major Concepts

Conflict

Conflict is a process which encompasses any interaction between two parties that is initiated by experiencing frustration. The expression of conflict may assume many forms, ranging from intellectual differences to physical violence.

Conflict Dyad

A conflict dyad consists of two social units. A social unit can be individuals, groups, or organizations. The concept "party and other" is synonymous with conflict dyad.

Conflict Episode

A conflict episode is a chain of five main "events" which occur when party and other disagree over an issue. The five main events of a conflict episode are: frustration, conceptualization, behavior, other's reactions, and outcome.

Frustration—The initial link in the chain of events is that, while actively engaged in an interaction, one party feels frustration. Frustration is an emotional reaction, actually present or anticipated, to the realization of one's goals. The perception of frustration stems from lack of satisfaction of "concerns" such as needs, desires, objectives, and standards of behavior, and initiates the conflict episode.

Conceptualization—The second link in the chain of events is conceptualization, or how the party experiencing frustration mentally processes the transpiring events. The party deals with the experienced frustration consciously, the party conceptualizes the problem situation. The party cognitively defines the conflict in terms of concerns of both parties along two "elements," defining the issue and salient alternatives.

Defining the Issue is the first element in a party's conceptualization of a conflict episode and involves assessment of the primary concerns of both parties. It may be accomplished egocentrically, insightfully, and/or with a sense of the size of the issue.

Salient alternatives is the second element of a party's conceptualization of the conflict situation. The party becomes aware of action alternatives to solve the conflict and their probable outcomes. Outcomes range from lose–lose to win–win possibilities. An exception is the either/or conceptualization which strives for a one party wins and the other loses outcome. An unresolvable situation occurs when neither party is willing or able to understand or cope with the defined issue.

Behavior—The third link in the chain of events behavior, is the result of party's mental processing of the situation. Behavior can be classified into five categories of orientations. Which orientation is chosen is dependent upon the relationship between party and other and how party wishes the relationship to be affected at the end of the conflict.

Orientation/desired result is defined as party's type of behavior on the basis of the degree to which party would desire to satisfy personal concerns and also the degree to which party would desire to satisfy the concerns of other. There are five such orientations and desired results: accommodative/ appeasement, avoidant/neglect, collaborative/integration, competitive/domination, and sharing/compromise.

1. Accommodative/appeasement is defined as the type of orientation that is opposite of competitive. The individual neglects his or her concerns. Accommodative behavior involves giving in to other's wishes with some degree of self-sacrifice. This is considered cooperative, but unassertive. It can be used when preserving harmony is important or when collecting social credits for later. The preferred result is appeasement.

2. Avoidant/neglect is defined as the type of orientation that involves side-stepping the issue for diplomatic reasons, withdrawing from a threatening situation , or postponing confrontation until a better time. This creates a lose–lose situation through unassertive and uncooperative means. This approach may be appropriate when the other party is more powerful, or the issue is unimportant. It may be used when it is more appropriate to solve a problem or to reduce tension and gain composure. The result of avoidant behavior is neglect.

3. Collaborative/integration is defined as the type of orientation which is assertive and cooperative. It is the opposite of avoidant behavior. It involves working with an individual in an attempt to identify a

solution and exploring insights to determine different viewpoints as related to conflict situations for the purpose of creatively solving the problem. This is a win–win strategy. The problem-solving process is utilized, but it sometimes takes more time than the results are worth. The result of collaboration is integration.

4. Competitive/domination is defined as a power orientation that is assertive and uncooperative. In competition, party is aggressive and pursues goals at other's expense. Competition results in the creation of a win–lose situation. This behavior can be appropriate if an unpopular decision must be made. If used excessively, party and/or other become afraid to admit mistakes. The result of competitive behavior is domination.

5. Sharing/compromise is defined as the type of orientation that is between domination and appeasement. It involves moderate yet incomplete satisfaction for both parties. The party must give up something but gets to keep something. The preferred result of sharing is compromise.

Strategic Objective is what party determines is feasible in "dimensions" of integration (total amount of satisfaction for both parties) and distribution (proportion of satisfaction going to each party). The strategic objective is the interaction of feasibility, orientations, and party's preferred end result.

Tactical Behavior is the use of specific maneuvers to achieve the desired integrative and distributive dimensions of party and other satisfaction.

Interaction/Reaction—The fourth link in the chain of events is interaction/reaction. This is defined as a feedback loop between behavior and conceptualization for both party and other. Escalation or de-escalation of the conflict results from the cycling of conceptualization, behavior, and interaction. Some "dynamics" which influence whether escalation or de-escalation occurs are revaluation, self-fulfilling prophesy, bias, communication breakdown, distrust, and resolution orientation. There are two types of interaction—the reactive aspect termed escalation/de-escalation and the self-conscious efforts of conflict management.

Escalation usually is defined as an increase in the level of conflict. Escalation behaviors may include increasing hostility between parties, increasing competitiveness, or using coercive tactics. De-escalation is defined as a decrease in the level of conflict during negotiations. Conflict management is defined as self-conscious strategies of the parties to manage the conflict between them.

Outcome is defined as the final link in the chain of events in the process model. This is the consequence of the aftermath of conflict which can be short- or long-term. Whether the outcome is viewed positively or negatively by party or other or by both depends upon what has transpired while reaching the outcome. Also, if residual frustration remains, conflict will come up again in the same or some other form when another issue arises. This is also the time when interaction between party and other ceases, some agreement has been made, or an agreement was made to let the issue drop.

Conflict aftermath is defined as the residual emotions after the agreement has been reached—emotions such as hostility or mistrust or warmth and trust. Elements of conflict aftermath set the climate for subsequent episodes between the two parties.

Long-term effects refers to a more long-range view of examining the outcomes of party's behavior with respect to other's goal achievement.

Third Party Intervention—third party intervention is the use of "process intervention" by a person not involved in the conflict in order to reach an outcome of the conflict situation. Process intervention includes: collaboration, de-escalation, and confrontation.

1. *Collaboration*—a joint integrative approach to reaching a desired state of affairs for the parties involved and for the organization. Collaboration is a frequent goal of the third party's efforts.
2. *De-escalation*—a method whereby the third party attempts to resolve the conflict by emphasizing the costs of continued competition or reopening communication between the two parties. The third party acts as a mediator.
3. *Confrontation*—a tactic in which the third party increases both parties' perceptions of the stakes in the conflict. This method attempts to elicit more assertive behavior from both parties. The eventual goal is to achieve collaboration after the main issue has been confronted.

Examples of Concepts Relevant to Role Practice

The nursing staff level at Sweetwater General Hospital is slightly below optimum. Rather than increase full-time staff, the hospital has regular float nurses who are cross-trained to fill in on specific units as the need arises. The system works well, except when more than one unit requires the services of the same float nurse. Then the one or more units who do not get the float nurse are left understaffed. Feelings of frustration are generated in the underserved units.

The situation is especially tense on the seventh floor, which consists of an MICU, SICU, and step down unit. Each head nurse constantly seeks to engage the services of the float nurse for her unit. Each of the three involved head nurses thinks the other two just want the float nurse to ease the case loads for their staff nurses (conceptualization). As the rivalry increases all the seventh floor head nurses try for the assignment of the float nurse (competitive behavior orientation). Each head nurse's strategic objective is to outdo the others in obtaining float nurse services.

The interpersonal relations among the seventh floor head nurses is deteriorating. There is pettiness, even open hostility (escalating interactions). In this unpleasant, highly competitive atmosphere, no one is attempting conflict management to defuse the situation. Staff nurses are seriously thinking of quitting or are asking to be transferred off the seventh floor. Before patient care can be negatively impacted, the Director of Nursing requests that a consultant be sent from corporate headquarters (third party intervention) to work with the conflict situation.

Following an assessment of the situation, the nurse consultant decides that each of the Head Nurses is sensing frustration when not obtaining the services of the float nurse because there are no guidelines by which all can agree on the appropriate assignment of the float nurses. She determines that a committee of all the head nurses should be formed. This committee would select its own leadership and operating procedures. It would be made clear that all head nurses would work with each other (confrontation) to develop the necessary guidelines. It was also made clear that the final product would be a set of guidelines which, when applied, would unequivocally determine assignment of the float nurses to the most needy units (de-escalation).

Ultimately the conflict situation would be resolved through changing behavior orientation from competitive to collaborative during the development of the guidelines. The trigger mechanism of conflict (frustration) would be removed through application of the guidelines.

Major Relational Statements

The process model of dyadic conflict developed by Thomas (1976) for his conflict theory is described in the following relational statements. This section is designed to illustrate how the major concepts are related to one another.

1. Conflict results from the perception that satisfaction of party's concerns is frustrated by other.
2. Conflict requires not a single event but five main events in a series of episodes.
3. Orientation to concern for other determines individual behavior.
4. Escalation/de-escalation follows the course of party's interaction with other.
5. Outcome of conflict involves an aftermath and long-term effects.
6. Third party intervention approaches conflict resolution through instigation of collaboration.

IMPLICATIONS OF THOMAS' CONFLICT THEORY FOR ROLE PRACTICE

Conflict theory is a useful theory for guiding the practice of nursing roles in practice settings. This section presents factors and methods of assessing, problem definition, plan implementation, and evaluation.

Factors to be Assessed and Methods of Assessing

The assessor or the third party intervener would, within the framework of a set of diagnostic questions derived by Thomas from his process model, establish that conflict exists. The diagnostic questions are not a part of the theory per se but derive from the dynamics of the theory. The first set of diagnostic questions seeks to identify whether or not party and other perceived loss or a threat of loss. Once frustration has been established, the third party intervener, through information obtained from the answers to the diagnostic questions, would seek to determine how party and other define the issue giving rise to frustration. The most common issues are listed earlier in this chapter.

The third party intervener would also determine from a second set of diagnostic questions which, if any, salient alternatives the party and other are considering for each other. The third party intervener would then determine from the third set of diagnostic questions which conflict handling orientations are being used by party and other. The next set of diagnostic questions would be utilized to determine how parties are interacting with each other and whether they are moving toward escalation or de-escalation.

The final set of diagnostic questions would attempt to determine the short-term and long-term outcomes of the existing conflict; most importantly answering the question, what effect will the current episode have on future episodes. In the process of obtaining answers to the diagnostic questions, the third party intervener incidentally learns if the conflict is either escalating or de-escalating. Methods used to obtain answers to the diagnostic questions would consist of direct observation of party and other's interactions, interviews with party and other, and reviewing documents that reflect or record data that would validate or negate information obtained from party and other.

Theory-Specific Problem Defining

The assessment data are sorted to identify the problems relative to the situation. The third party intervener selects the most salient problem from the problems identified. La Monica (1990) states, "a clearly stated problem structures the whole problem-solving process because what has to be done to solve the problem and evaluate outcomes becomes apparent only when the problem statement is clear and specific (p. 12)." To assist in problem-defining, La Monica's (1990) technique is to identify the difference between the actual prevailing conditions and the desired state of conditions.

Thomas' theory directs the third party intervener to validate the presence of frustration and identify its source. The problem statement then becomes a statement of the difference between the actual and the optimal state of the most salient issue of the conflict. La Monica's formulation as applied to Thomas' Conflict Theory would direct the third party intervener to determine what issue in the prevailing conditions is causing party or other to experience frustration. Once the issue is determined, its optimal state is described. The nature of the difference between the two states defines the specific source of frustration.

Problem Resolution Plan

Planning is the third step in the problem-solving approach. The interventions available to the third party intervener, according to Thomas (1976), are confrontation, de-escalation, and collaboration. To achieve the ultimate goal, conflict resolution, the third party intervener arranges for party and other to come together to confront their contentious issues. The purpose of such a meeting is to afford the third party intervener an opportunity to point out to party and other the disadvantages of their current conflict-handling orientation. Once party and other came to understand how counterproductive their interactions are, de-escalation may spontaneously occur. If not, the third party intervener develops an agenda which directs party and other to a collaborative approach to solve their problems and resolve their conflict.

Implementation of the Plan

The fourth step in the problem-solving approach is implementing or putting the plan into operation. The confrontation meeting is convened as planned. The third party intervener chairs the confrontation meeting and monitors the coming together of all parties to the conflict. As the differences are aired, the negatives of conflict are pointed out, and the positives of conflict resolution are emphasized. Once the majority of the parties to the conflict indicate they are convinced resolution is desirable, the third party intervener takes a more passive role while party and other collaboratively move toward conflict resolution.

Evaluation of the Plan

The problem-solving process is complete when the process and outcome evaluation is accomplished. Outcome evaluation is the determination that frustration is sufficiently reduced to allow de-escalation to the point of conflict resolution to occur. Process evaluation measures the extent the substantive input of the third party intervener has influenced the resolution of the conflict through bringing party and other into the collaborative orientation so they can resolve their frustrating issue. Some approaches to process evaluation might include completion of evaluation forms, scores on evaluation instruments, or observational feedback.

THEORY-DIRECTED ROLE PRACTICE FOR THE FOGRAM HOSPITAL CASE

The problem-solving process and Thomas' (1976) conflict theory are used simultaneously to alleviate the problem demonstrated in the FGH case. This application of theory within the framework of the problem-solving process represents a systematic theoretical resolution of a problem.

Assessing

In preparation for third party intervention, the intervener prepares the diagnostic questions specific for the FGH situation. These and the data obtained are depicted in Table 10.2.

Table 10.2　Assessment questions and relevant case data

Key Questions	Relevant Data
1. *Who* experiences *what* frustration?	Nursing staff: Routine procedures not performed, such as temperatures, I & Os. Dietary department: Disruption of breakfast service. Payroll department: Inaccurate work records. Admission department: Inaccurate patient counts as well as misinformation on bed availability. Patient billing: Inaccurate reports of drug, equipment, and supply usage. Pharmacy, Central Supply, Laundry: Disruption of replacement system.
2. How do party and other perceive the situation?	All parties' perceptions lack accuracy and movement toward resolution.
3. How are party and other dealing with each other?	All parties behaving in the competitive (domination) conflict-handling orientation.
4. What is the effect of party and other's interactions?	Escalation of conflict.
5. Without intervention what is the short-term trajectory and long-term trajectory of events?	Further escalation with deteriorating relations and long-term residual hostility.

The third party intervener also observes the normal flow of activities of FGH and reviews records (charts, incident reports, and departmental memos, for example). Additionally, physicians, patients, and their visitors are interviewed.

Problem Defining

From the accumulated data the third party intervener identifies a number of interdepartmental frustrations, thereby establishing that conflict exists. These data also provide information that help the third party intervener determine what is the problem. To frame the problem statement the La Monica technique of contrasting the actual and optimal states is applied. The La Monica (1990) technique applied to problem defining in the FGH case is as follows:

Actual: Archaic procedures in an upgraded hospital setting.

Optimal: Updated procedures congruent with an upgraded hospital setting.

Problem: Present hospital personnel experiencing frustration leading to conflict attempting to function under current FGH operating procedures.

Planning

Identifying the goal to be achieved initiates the planning process. Since the problem centers on FGH's personnel's inability to operate effectively under FGH's current procedures, the goal is to have hospital personnel (night nurses [party] and articulating groups [other]) functioning without frustration and subsequent conflict under updated FGH operating procedures.

From the assessment data it is clear that the conflict is widespread and escalating. The third party intervener now knows that the dyad of night nurses and numerous articulating groups is involved and to bring them all together at the same time on more than one occasion requires powerful administrative support. Therefore, planning begins with requesting assurance from nursing and hospital administration that representation at and participation in the third party intervener meetings is mandatory.

Past experience helps the third party intervener estimate the length and number of sessions needed. The agenda for the first session is developed to start the participants confronting their frustrations. Subsequent agendas are developed based on what has transpired in the previous session. The third party intervener maintains control of the sessions for several reasons:

1. to keep the group focused on the confrontation purpose
2. to prevent derailing of the intervention plan
3. to provide leadership until natural leaders emerge from the group
4. to maintain calm and order in a potentially explosive situation.

At some point during a confrontation session the third party intervener will identify the group's readiness to convert to the collaborative mode. At this time an agenda is developed which prepares the group to assume greater responsibility for managing the sessions, focussing on the causes of their frustration and conflict, and generating recommendations for solution to FGH's dilemma.

Implementing

To begin the first confrontational meeting, the third party intervener establishes an open environment conducive to the airing of grievances. As members voice their experiences, they are allowed to express emotion, even hostility, but abusiveness is not permitted.

Listening to the night nurses and departmental representatives (party and other) air their grievances allows the third party intervener to reconstruct the conflict episodes. The major frustration expressed by all parties is inability to attain personal standards of job performance. Further, all parties assess the issue egocentrically; that is, solely in the light of their own concerns. From determining which salient alternatives party and other are using, the third party intervener can only recognize a win for party and lose for other choice in use.

The behaviors exhibited during the conflict episodes most frequently are of the competitive orientation, with the expected result that party's position would prevail (dominate) over other's. The strategic object of party saw little feasibility in obtaining much satisfaction for distribution between self and other in the current situation. Therefore, the only tactical behaviors employed were argument and spiteful acts.

During each episode, party and other's interactions and reactions escalated as they recycled their unaltered conceptualizations without any attempt at conflict management. The outcome was periods of truce interspersed with conflict episodes. Without intervention the conflict between party and other will go on indefinitely.

While the agenda for the confrontation meeting is followed and members are expressing themselves, the third party intervener listens carefully for opportunities to point out destructive or constructive points made by the speakers. This tactic is continued throughout the first and subsequent meetings until the third party intervener determines the group is ready to move into a collaborative posture.

The collaborative phase begins with some instruction on how to function collaboratively, assurance of administrative support for resources and, ultimately, outcome of the group's efforts. The group is directed to choose its own leadership and set its own agendas. The third party intervener suggests and encourages but does not totally relinquish control of the group.

At first the collaborative sessions progress tentatively as party and other work through the aftermath of their shared conflict. Gradually, thinking shifts from they and them to we and us. Personality issues fade as the real issues surface. Party and other then settle down to developing hospital-wide procedures which will promote efficiency and harmonious relations among the personnel at FGH. All the problems at FGH may not be solved, but conditions are improving and personnel are using collaboration to achieve resolution of conflict.

Evaluating

Outcome evaluation is based upon the identified goal. The goal for the FGH case situation was stated as: Present hospital personnel functioning without frustration under updated FGH procedures. Evidence that the goal was achieved involves determining that frustration is markedly reduced or absent. In the FGH case, as realization that party and other were dealing with the cause of the many disruptions and inaccuracies and their consequences, the arguing, blaming, and pettiness diminished. With the institution of more congruent procedures, morale improved. The reduction or absence of frustration was also validated through interviews between the third party intervener and a sampling of hospital personnel.

In process evaluation the third party intervener measures the efficiency of the intervention tactics employed. Feedback, in the form of written and oral evaluation, is obtained from the departmental representatives on the management of meetings, agendas for meetings, and direction for initiating and conducting the collaborative effort. Evaluation of the consultation by the administration of FGH is presented on Kutani Megaconglomerate Incorporated's official evaluation form.

SUMMARY

Thomas' conflict theory was used to demonstrate how nurses can resolve conflict situations in the work setting. Also illustrated was how the concepts of the theory drive the problem-solving process, leading to logical and coherent problem resolution.

A review of nursing literature reveals consistent use of the Thomas conflict theory as an appropriate approach to conflict management. Barton's (1991) report on a study of Thomas' conflict management behaviors found that compromise was the behavior of choice by the majority of the nurses in the study. *Nursing 85* and *Nursing 86* published a series of articles by Huttman

(1985), Isaac (1985), Bruha (1986), and Isaac (1986) demonstrating how Thomas' preferred conflict management behavior of collaboration can be achieved.

REFERENCES

Barton, A. (1991). Conflict resolution by nurse managers. *Nursing Management, 4*(2), 14–15.

Bruha, S. (1986). You can conquer conflict. *Nursing 86, 16*(1), 81–83.

Corwin, R. (1969). Patterns of organizational conflict. *Administrative Science Quarterly, 14,* 507–521.

Filley, A. (1975). *Interpersonal conflict resolution.* Morristown, NJ: Scott Foresman.

Huttman, B. (1985). The way to go—from conflict to collegiality. *Nursing 85, 15*(4), 89–92.

Isaac, S. (1985). Conflict—why don't you get along with that co-worker. *Nursing 85, 15*(12), 65–67.

Issac, S. (1986). 5 ways to resolve conflict. *Nursing 86, 16*(3), 89–91.

La Monica, E. L. (1990). *Management in nursing.* New York: Springer Publishing Co.

Pondy, L. R. (1967). Organizational conflict: Concepts and models. *Administrative Science Quarterly, 12,* 296–320.

Thomas, K. (1976). Conflict and conflict management. In M. D. Dunnette (Ed.) *Handbook of industrial and organizational psychology* (pp. 889–935). Chicago: Rand McNally.

SUGGESTED READINGS

Filley, A. (1980). Types and sources of conflict, In M. Berger, D. Elhart, S. Firsich, & S. Jordan (Eds.) *Management for nurses: A multidisciplinary approach.* St. Louis: C. V. Mosby.

Pondy, L. R. (1966). A systems theory of organizational conflict. *Academy of Management Journal. 9*(3), 246–256.

Pondy, L. R. (1969). Variances of organizational conflict. *Administrative Science Quarterly. 14,* 449–506.

Chapter 11

Strategy for Theory-Directed Nursing Practice

Shirley Melat Ziegler

METHODOLOGY FOR DELIVERY OF NURSING CARE

Nursing care is delivered using one of two processes—nursing process and the problem-solving process. Process is defined in the dictionary as a particular method of doing something, generally involving a number of steps or operations. In direct client care this process is popularly called the nursing process. In selected nursing roles, such as the nurse administrator, the process is popularly termed problem-solving. Both processes involve critical thinking. Nursing process is described first.

The Nursing Process

Although there is no consensus in nursing regarding the steps of the nursing process, five steps are described in this book. The interrelationships among the steps reflect the Nursing Process Model described by Ziegler, Vaughan-Wrobel, and Erlen (1986). In this model each step of the nursing process is regarded as a process ending in a product. In this book the gerund (a verbal noun ending in "ing") is used when the step is viewed as a process. The noun is used when the step is viewed as a product. For example, diagnos*ing* is used when the second step of the nursing process is viewed as a process; diagnos*is* is used when the second step is viewed as a product.

Steps of the Nursing Process Model

The five steps of the nursing process are defined as follows (Ziegler et al., 1986):

- *Assessing,* the first step of the nursing process, is defined as the act of systematically collecting and organizing information to determine a client's need for nursing care. Assessment data are the product of assessing.
- *Diagnosing,* the second step, is defined as arriving at a judgment or conclusion about the client from data obtained during the assessing step. Nursing diagnosis is the product of diagnosing.
- *Planning,* the third step, is defined as determining the plan for implementing the client's need for nursing care. The nursing care plan is the product of planning.
- *Implementing,* the fourth step, is defined as executing or carrying out the planned nursing interventions. Implementation is the product of implementing and is evidenced by documentation on the client's record.
- *Evaluating,* the last step, is defined as judging the efficacy of nursing interventions. Evaluation is the product of evaluating.

A glossary of the terms used in the Nursing Process Model is provided in Appendix A.

Interrelationships Among the Steps of the Nursing Process Model

The interrelationships among the steps are illustrated in Figure 11.1. Several of the steps consist of a number of components (substeps). The components of the steps are presented in Figure 11.2 as well as the interrelationships among the components in the steps.

Assessing/Assessment. The purpose of assessing is to generate nursing diagnoses. The assessment data consists of subjective and objective data. *Subjective data* consists of information that the client actually tells the nurse

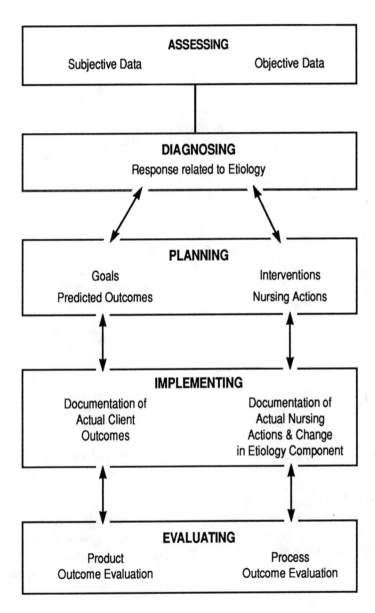

Figure 11.1 Interrelationships among the steps of the Nursing Process Model.

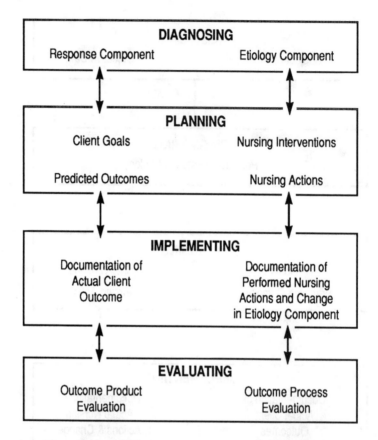

The response component is reassessed. The current client response (actual client outcome) is compared to the predicted client outcomes and the extent that the response is actually modified in the direction predicted is evaluated.

The completed nursing actions are documented and compared against the planned nursing actions. The extent that the planned actions were completed is evaluated.

The etiology component is reassessed and documented. The extent that the etiology is actually modified is evaluated.

Figure 11.2 Components of the steps of the Nursing Process Model and interrelationships among the steps.

during assessing. In the subjective data realm the client is the expert. Subjective data is also referred to as "symptoms." *Objective data* consists of information obtained by the nurse's observations. In the objective data realm the nurse is the expert. Objective data is also referred to as "signs." In addition, objective data may consist of observations made by other members of the health team. For example, the client's chart contains objective data observed by various members of the health team. Without assessment data, there is nothing upon which to base the nursing diagnosis statements.

Diagnosing/Diagnoses. Diagnosing is the pivotal step of the nursing process and is supported by subjective and objective assessment data. The product of diagnosing—the nursing diagnosis statement—consists of two components. The first component is the client's potential or actual unhealthful response. The second component is the hypothesized cause or etiology for the response.

A potential client response is a prediction that certain unhealthful client responses are probable in the future. This prediction is based on the nurse's observation of the presence of certain risk factors that theory links with the unhealthful response. An actual unhealthful client response is a client behavior observed by the nurse which is compared against theoretical norms and then judged unhealthful.

The etiology component of the nursing diagnosis statement is the hypothesized cause of the client's actual or potentially unhealthful response. Causation is recognized as multiple in nature. The cause, selected by the nurse as the etiology component, is one that is amenable to independent nursing actions; that is, the etiology is one of the causative variables over which nursing has direct control. Additionally, the variable is believed to be a major causative factor of the client's actual or potential unhealthful response. "The goal of using etiology in clinical nursing practice is to make nursing diagnostic statements descriptive of the patient and prescriptive of the nursing interventions that the patient requires" (Miller, 1989, p. 39).

Because of the pivotal role the nursing diagnosis statement plays in the nursing process, the critical characteristics of the diagnosis statement are presented in Table 11.1. (Ziegler et al., 1986). Fourteen characteristics are identified: four general characteristics for the diagnosis statement as product; four for the response component; four for the etiology component; and two for the process of diagnosing. These characteristics can be used to guide the generation of nursing diagnoses and to evaluate the quality of the nursing diagnoses so generated.

Planning/Plan. Planning, the third step of the nursing process, is directed by the nursing diagnosis statement. Without this statement there is nothing

Table 11.1 Characteristics of Nursing Diagnosis*

Component	Characteristic
Product: General	1. Both the response and etiology component are present 2. The components are joined with a "related-to" phrase 3. The response component is written first and the etiology component is written second 4. The statement is asymmetrical, not circular
Response Component	5. The response is clearly unhealthy or written as a potentially unhealthful response 6. Only one response is identified for each diagnosis statement 7. The response has the potential for modification 8. The response is concrete enough to generate specific client goals
Etiology Component	9. Only one etiology is identified for each diagnosis statement 10. The etiology is potentially changeable 11. The activity requiring modification is within the boundaries of nursing's independent functions; nurse is capable, and is legally and ethically expected to treat 12. Etiology is concrete enough to generate specific nursing interventions
Process	13. Evidence that a pattern exists in the assessment data upon which the diagnosis was made (including both subjective and objective data) 14. Evidence that the client's response is related to the etiology (cause) including both empirical and theoretical evidence

*Reprinted from Ziegler, S. M., Vaughan-Wrobel, B. & Erlen, J. (1986). *Nursing Process, Nursing Diagnosis, Nursing Knowledge: Avenues to Autonomy*, (p. 90). Norwalk, CT: Appleton-Century-Crofts.

upon which to base the nursing care plan. Because of the role the nursing diagnosis statement plays in planning and implementing nursing care, diagnosing is considered the pivotal step of the nursing process.

The nursing care plan is generated from the nursing diagnosis statement and consists of four components—client goal, predicted client outcomes, nursing interventions, and nursing actions. The client goal and predicted client outcomes are generated from the response component of the nursing diagnosis statement. The nursing interventions and nursing actions are generated from the etiology component of the nursing diagnosis statement.

The client goal is the desired client response stated in the direction of health. The client goal is stated in abstract terms and is standard for a given client response. The goal is individualized to the client in the client predicted outcomes.

Client predicted outcomes consist of time-specific and measurable client responses the nurse expects to observe after nursing interventions and actions have been implemented. Client predicted outcomes are unique to the client in that they are realistic expectations for this particular client. These expectations are based on client data. Thus, they identify a change in the subjective and objective data used to support the response component of the nursing diagnosis statement.

Nursing interventions are nursing acts that prevent, modify, remove, or control the variable(s) causing the client's potential or actual unhealthful response. Thus, nursing interventions are etiology-directed. The nursing interventions are the means used by the nurse to help the client to achieve the goal and predicted outcomes. Interventions are highly abstract and are standard for the etiology. For example, if the etiology is "lack of knowledge . . .", the nursing intervention is "teach the client . . .". Nursing interventions are individualized for each client through the specific nursing actions.

Nursing actions are the time-specific and documentable activities planned by the nurse to implement the nursing interventions. They are individualized to the client. Nursing actions are unique for the client in that they are based on assessment data and the special characteristics of the client. Without a nursing care plan there is nothing upon which to base systematic nursing care.

Implementing/Implementation. During the implementing step the nurse provides the planned nursing care to the client. Following implementation, the nurse's actions are documented. Observed change in the response and in the etiology components of the nursing diagnosis statement are also documented. If the care plan is not implemented and documented, there is nothing upon which to base the last step of the nursing process—evaluating.

Evaluating/Evaluation. After the care plan is implemented and the nurse's actions and the observed change in the response and etiology components of the nursing diagnosis are documented, evaluating is initiated. The documentation is the basis of evaluation. Evaluation consists of two components—outcome product evaluation and outcome process evaluation.

Outcome product evaluation involves making a judgment about the degree to which the client goal(s) have been achieved; the documented client outcomes are compared to the predicted client outcomes. The degree to which predicted client outcomes are achieved is judged and documented. This documentation forms the basis for nursing accountability for the quality of nursing care.

Outcome process evaluation is composed of two parts—one focused on the nurse, the other focused on the client. Outcome process evaluation, when focused on the nurse, involves making a judgment regarding the extent that planned nursing actions were actually implemented. It is generated from a comparison of the planned nursing actions and the documented activities of the nurse. Outcome process evaluation, when focused on the client, involves making a judgment regarding the extent that planned nursing actions are successful in modifying the etiology. It is generated from a comparison of the etiology component before and after nursing actions are documented. It should reflect a change in the subjective and objective data used to support the etiology component of the nursing diagnosis statement. For example, if the etiology component was "lack of knowledge," the knowledge level of the client would be evaluated after the nursing intervention of teaching had occurred.

Evaluation cannot take place without a nursing diagnosis statement (based on assessment data), a nursing care plan (directed by the nursing diagnosis statement), and nursing care delivery (directed by the nursing care plan). The five steps of the nursing process are, thus, highly interrelated.

The Problem-Solving Method

Like the nursing process, the number of steps in the problem-solving process and the interrelationship among the steps vary according to author. In nursing literature problem solving is sometimes equated with the nursing process. Both La Monica (1990) and Burns and Grove (1987) presented comparisons between the nursing process and basic problem solving. This book uses a composite of these two conceptualizations. Thus, the problem-solving process used in this book is conceptualized as consisting of five steps: assessing, problem defining, planning, implementing, and evaluating.

The products of these five steps are: assessment, problem, plan, implementation, and evaluation.

Assessing/Assessment

In this book the first step of problem solving is termed assessing. The name for the first step of the problem-solving process varies in the literature. La Monica (1990) used the term problem-solving problem identification. "A problem is identified by the difference between what is actually happening (the actual) in a situation and what one wishes to have occur (the optimal)" (La Monica, 1990, p. 11). In order to identify a problem area, one gathers and examines data relevant to the situation. In contrast, Burns and Grove (1987) named the first step data collection.

Problem Defining/Problem

The second step of problem solving is termed problem defining. Problem defining results in a problem statement which is a negative statement describing the condition in the situation considered unacceptable and in need of change. Although it is not generally stated in a two-component statement, as is a nursing diagnosis, the hypothesized cause of the problem is implicit. The problem may be "caused" by multiple factors. "Acknowledging these factors (causes) will allow a problem to be broken down into manageable proportions" (TNA Professional Services Committee, 1983, p. 9). Although La Monica (1990) places the determination of why the problem exists under a step she terms "problem analysis," she concurs that both the problem and its cause must be identified.

Planning/Plan

The third step of problem solving is termed planning. Unlike the planning step in the nursing process, goals and interventions have not been traditionally cited as components of planning. They are, however, implicit components. Thus, Burns and Grove (1987) included goal setting and the identification of solutions as components of the planning step. A goal is simply a restated problem (La Monica, 1990). A problem statement is the negative statement in that it addresses a condition that is unacceptable. A goal addresses the unacceptable in a positive statement; that is, it states the condition of acceptability.

Identifying solutions to the problem involves determining the strategies that have potential for solving the problem and achieving the goal. These strategies are "directed toward resolving or ameliorating the actual factors [causes] that impinge on the situation" (TNA Professional Services Committee, 1983, p. 9).

Implementing/Implementation

Implementing involves carrying out the plan of action. The action is documented and the documentation guides the evaluating step of the problem-solving process.

Evaluating/Evaluation

As in the evaluating step of nursing process, evaluating both the nursing actions to achieve the goals (outcome process evaluation) and the situational outcomes of the actions (outcome product evaluation) is important. Perhaps the actions were never implemented due to unforeseen circumstances. If actions were implemented, the outcomes achieved are observed and compared to the goals to determine the effectiveness of the problem-solving process.

Both problem solving and nursing process are abstract processes which require critical thinking and complex reasoning. Implementation of the steps of the two processes is not automatic or a rote application of steps. The problem-solving process and the nursing process are viewed as the methodology for the delivery of nursing care. Through application of scientific theory to this process, quality care is provided.

SCIENTIFIC THEORY FOR PRACTICE

Definitions of the theoretical terms used in this book are provided. The processes of theory formalization and identification of a theory's implications for practice are described.

Theoretical Terms

To facilitate the reader's understanding, Appendix B contains a glossary of theory terms used in this book. Scientific theory is defined "a set of interrelated constructs [concepts], definitions, and propositions that present a systematic view of phenomena by specifying relations among concepts, with the purpose of explaining and predicting the phenomena" (Kerlinger, 1973, p. 9). The two major terms used in this definition (concepts and propositions) are further explicated.

Concept

A concept is a term used to express a mental image of some object or event in the real world (Zetterberg, 1965). Concepts are "ideas about classes of ideas derived from experience and expressed through symbols" (Bloom, 1975, p. 37). "Concepts indicate the subject matter of a theory" Jacox, 1992, p. 351). "Variables are the empirical characteristics of concepts that can take on different degrees" (Bloom, 1975, p. 43). Concepts are not observed directly, but are associated with empirical indicators. Empirical indicators are behavioral observations that can be made in the real world utilizing one or more of the five senses. Some authors use the term empirical referent for empirical indicators. "Empirical referents are defined as classes or categories of actual events which by their existence or presence demonstrate the occurrence of the concept" (Walker & Avant, 1988, p. 43).

Proposition

"When two or more concepts are joined together (related) they are wed; they have become a proposition" (Bloom, 1975, p. 44). A proposition is a statement stating how two or more concepts of a theory are related. Propositions that link two or more concepts are called relational statements. It is the relational statements making up a theory that provide the basis of prediction and explanation in practice.

Theories are, by their very nature, highly abstract. To be useful in nursing they need to be placed into a format useful to the nurse in practice. The format is summarized in Table 11.2 and described in the following section.

THEORY FORMALIZATION

Theory formalization "identifies the concepts, definitions, and propositions that make up a theory" (Fawcett & Downs, 1986, p. 15). The steps in theory formalization used in this book are:

1. Name the theory and theorist.
2. Identify the focus of the theory the phenomenon or clinical event addressed).
3. Name the major concepts of the theory.
4. Identify the theoretical definitions of the major concepts.
5. Generate concrete examples of concepts that are familiar to nurses in practice.
6. Identify the major relational statements/assumptions.

Table 11.2   Developing a Theory for Practice

Theory Formalization

1.	Name of theory and theorist
2.	Focus of theory or phenomenon addressed
3.	Major concepts
4.	Theoretical definitions of major concepts
5.	Concrete examples of concepts that are familiar to nurses in practice
6.	Major relational statements/assumptions

Research Support for the Theory	
7.	Review research literature
8.	Evaluate the level of empirical support for the theory

Implications for Practice	
9.	Factors (concepts, variables) to be assessed
10.	Methods of assessing
11.	Norms for responses/problems
12.	Theory-specific diagnoses/problems: relational statements that factor A (response) is caused, at least in part, by factor B.
13.	Theory-specific interventions: Relational statements that factor B is modified by factor C.

Many theories used by nurses can be identified by name and by the theorist or theorists that generated and developed the theory. Nurses need to be able to identify the generator of a theory because access to the literature regarding the theory is frequently through the author's name.

The focus of the theory, that is, that part of clinical practice which the theory describes, predicts, explains, and gives an understanding of, is identified. What specific clinical or health care setting problem does the theory address? For example, does the theory address pain, crisis, adaptation, coping, or some other phenomenon? The theories selected to demonstrate the strategy for theory-directed nursing practice in this book describe and explain the phenomena of crisis, teaching-learning, depression, family functioning, psychosocial development, coping with stress, anxiety, change, and conflict.

RESEARCH SUPPORT FOR THE THEORY

The amount of empirical support that exists for the theory is determined by conducting a review of the literature. A summary of literature is generated. A judgment is made regarding whether or not adequate research support is available. If the level of research support for the theory is deemed adequate, the theory's implications for practice are derived. This step in theory formalization is not demonstrated in this book because the demonstration chapters do not include a literature review due to space restrictions. However, no theory should be utilized by the nurse that has not received at least some empirical support through research.

IMPLICATIONS FOR PRACTICE

The steps in deriving the theory's implications for practice are:

1. Identify the factors to be assessed.
2. Identify the methods of assessing.
3. Identify the standards/norms for responses.
4. Identify theory-specific diagnoses/problems: Relational statements that concept/variable A (response) is caused at least in part, by concept/variable B.
5. Generate theory-specific interventions: Relational statements that concept/variable B is modified by concept/variable C.

Based on the major concepts of the theory, the concepts/variables in the client or nursing situation that are to be assessed are identified. It is these empirical indicators of the theory's concepts that make up the variables to be assessed. Methods to assess these variables are described. The behavioral norms for the concepts described in the theory are listed. For example, if anxiety is being assessed, the level of the client's anxiety is compared to normal anxiety levels. Based on the relational statements, theory-specific diagnoses/problems are identified. The relational statements assert that variable A (client response or nursing situation) is caused, at least in part, by variable B. Theory-specific interventions are deduced. Relational statements again provide the basis for predicting that variable B (the causative variable) may be modified by implementing variable C (the intervention variable).

STRATEGY FOR THEORY-DIRECTED NURSING PRACTICE

The format for identifying the implications of a theory for practice is interfaced with the steps of the nursing process and problem-solving process described earlier. Work sheets for planning theory-directed nursing practice are presented in Figure 11.3. (Nursing Process) and Figure 11.4. (Problem-Solving Process).

Assessing

In the first step of the process, assessing, theory is used to provide structure and direction for the assessment. Theory guides the selection of the characteristics of the client and/or situation to be observed. The concepts and relational statements of the theory name, describe, and explain these characteristics to be assessed. In this book, the authors of Chapter 5 explicitly illustrate this link by providing a guide for assessing family functioning using Bowen's theory. The theoretical basis for collecting specific data are provided.

Research is needed to validate the description and explanation of the phenomena offered by the theory. In addition, methodological research aids in the development of assessment instruments that are both valid and reliable; that is, the instrument measures what it claims to measure, and it measures that concept consistently and accurately. Baldwin's chapter illustrates the generation of assessing instruments based on theory by identifying the Jalowiec Coping Scale, a scale developed by nurses based on Lazarus' theory. Practice consists of psychomotor skills in the use of the assessment tools and cognitive skills in interpreting the data collected by these tools.

Without theory there is no rationale for collecting specific data. Without research there is no justification for considering a theory valid, nor are there valid and reliable tools to assess the characteristics of the client and or/situation. Without the use of theory in practice there is no scientific knowledge (theory) directing nursing care.

Diagnosing/Problem Defining

In the second step of the process, diagnosing/problem defining, theory is used in hypothesis formulation. "An hypothesis is a conjectural statement of the relation between two or more concepts" (Kerlinger, 1973, p. 18). Theory predicts a relationship among the observations made, provides the standards against which the client's responses or factors in a specific situation are compared, and is used to determine if the observed client responses fall

THEORETICAL FRAMEWORK

Assessment Data	

Nursing Diagnosis	
Response Component	Etiology Component
Subjective Data	Subjective Data
Objective Data	Objective Data

Plan	
Client Goal	Nursing Interventions
Predicted Outcomes	Nursing Actions

Evaluation	
Client Outcome	Process Outcome
	Nurse
	Client

Figure 11.3 Work sheet for theory-directed nursing practice: Nursing process.

THEORETICAL FRAMEWORK

Assessment Data

Identified Problem	
Problem	Implicit Cause
Subjective Data	Subjective Data
Objective Data	Objective Data

Plan	
Goal Setting	Identified Solutions
Predicted Outcomes	Planned Actions

Evaluation	
Actual Outcome	Process Outcome
	Nurse Cause / Situation

Figure 11.4 Work sheet for theory-directed nursing practice: Problem-solving process.

within an acceptable range of health or if the situation's factors appear to be acceptable. If not, a judgment is made that an unhealthful client response or problem situation exists. Theory is then used to guide the formulation of the causative variables for the undesirable client response or problem situation by asserting that certain responses or factors in a situation are caused by certain variables.

Evidence of these variables is sought by assessing for them. If the variables are present, a working hypothesis (the nursing diagnosis statement/problem statement) that asserts that a client/situation has a unhealthful response/ problem and that this response/problem is caused by the presence of certain other factors is made. Ideally, the relationship between a response/problem and a cause proposed in a theory has been supported by research.

Potential nursing diagnoses/problems are somewhat different because an undesirable response has not yet occurred. The theory guides the nurse to assess for the presence of certain variables believed to be related to undesirable responses/situations. These variables are frequently called risk factors. The presence of these risk factors are used to predict potential unhealthful/ undesirable responses/situations. For example, potential heart disease is diagnosed from the presence of elevated blood levels, a high fat diet, a sedentary lifestyle, and a family history of heart disease. The relationship among these variables has been demonstrated through research, and theory exists to explain this relationship.

Those theories most relevant for use in assessing and diagnosing/problem defining are those that address etiological variables which are manipulated by the nurse operating under the nursing professional license. Thus, diagnoses/ problems applicable to the independent role of the nurse are those in which the etiology is amenable to independent manipulation by the nurse. If the variables cannot be manipulated by the nurse independently, then referral may be appropriate, and/or the interdependent role is implemented. Thus, the diagnosis/problem statement is a working hypothesis, based on theory and supporting research, which asserts that response/problem A is caused, at least in part, by etiology B. This working hypothesis then forms the basis of the third step of the process—planning.

Planning

Theory is used in the third step of the process, planning, by providing the rationale for intervention. The nurse faces the question, "What can I do that would change or modify the cause so that the unhealthful, or potentially unhealthful, response/problem situation can be modified?" Thus, theory is used to predict that intervention C will modify the variables making up the etiology component of the statement. In turn, once the etiology is modified, the unhealthful response/problem situation will be modified. When nurses identify a nursing technique believed effective in modifying the variables making up the etiology component, they explicitly formulate a causal hypothesis. "Such a hypothesis predicts that certain kinds of means will produce certain kinds of effects under a given set of practice conditions" (Wooldridge, Leonard, & Skipper, 1983, p. 30).

Theory provides the basis of the nursing actions involved in intervening. For example, if the etiology of a diagnosis statement is that the client lacks sufficient knowledge, then a teaching-learning theory is needed to guide the intervention. In addition, developmental theory may be used to determine the type of teaching-learning intervention, that is, the nursing actions that are most appropriate.

Implementing

In the implementing step, the nurse carries out the theory-based plan. The nursing actions and the responses to the nursing actions are documented.

Evaluating

The purpose of evaluating is to judge the worth of a practice. Theory provides the standards against which outcomes are to be compared. In addition, evaluation models, which describe the evaluation process, give guidance to this last step of the process. For example, one evaluation model asserts that to determine the worth of a practice, one compares outcome data with clearly specified objectives reflected in predicted outcomes.

STRATEGY FOR THEORY-DIRECTED NURSING PRACTICE—AN ILLUSTRATION

Two phenomena are used to illustrate the linking of theory with the nursing problem-solving processes—life satisfaction in the elderly and infant colic.

Life Satisfaction in the Elderly

With lengthening life span, concern for the quality of life for older persons has been addressed by a number of disciplines. Activity theory, disengagement theory, and continuity theory have been proposed to explain the psychosocial aspects of successful aging (Burbank, 1986). Because these theories cite different etiologies for the same phenomena—life satisfaction in the elderly—the nursing diagnoses generated from these theories are different and the nursing interventions designed to treat the diagnoses are different.

Assessing

The phenomena that these theories address is life satisfaction in the elderly (Table 11.3). Life satisfaction can be defined as general psychological well-being and satisfaction with life. A number of assessment instruments have been developed to assess life satisfaction. Table 11.3 summarizes the three theories, which differ primarily in their explanation of the etiology of

Table 11.3   Summary of Psychological Theories of Life Satisfaction in the Elderly

Phenomena	Characteristics
Life satisfaction in the elderly (successful aging)	Degree one is presently content or pleased with general life situation. Includes taking pleasure from everyday activities and regarding one's life as meaningful.

Theory	Relational statements
Activity	Activity is positively associated with life satisfaction. Continued social role participation is necessary for positive adjustment to old age.
Disengagement	Disengagement (decreased interaction) is inevitable for all aging individuals. Disengagement (decreased interaction) of aging individuals from society is accompanied by the withdrawal of society from individuals. Disengagement (decreased interaction) is associated with successful aging.
Continuity	Personality remains consistent as age increases in normal men and women. Personality influences life satisfaction. Personality style is associated with both activity level and life satisfaction.

life satisfaction. Each theory provides a different structure and direction for the assessment. Thus, in activity theory, activity (action-oriented pursuits) is assessed. In disengagement theory, the degree of interaction between the aging client and society is assessed. In continuity theory, role activity (the extent and intensity of involvement in different social roles) and personality type are assessed, including the client's life-long activity preferences.

Diagnosing

The major relational statements from each theory are used to generate theory-specific diagnoses (Table 11.3). From activity theory, the diagnosis "low level of life satisfaction related to inadequate activity" could be generated. This diagnosis is generated from the statement that continued social role participation is necessary for positive adjustment to old age. From disengagement theory, a diagnosis could be "low level of life satisfaction related to inadequate disengagement." This diagnosis is generated from the relational statement: Disengagement (decreased interaction) is associated with successful aging. From continuity theory, a diagnosis could be "low level of life satisfaction related to a mismatch between personality and activity." This diagnosis is based on the relational statements that personality style is associated with both activity level and life satisfaction.

Planning

Goals and predicted outcomes are generated from the response component of the diagnosis—low level of life satisfaction. Interventions are generated from the theory-based etiology components of the diagnoses. Because the theories identify different etiologies, the interventions from the three theories are different. In activity theory, efforts are made to increase the activity level of the client. In disengagement theory, efforts are made to decrease the activity level of the client. In continuity theory, efforts are directed at matching the client's preferences for activity.

Implementing

The planned etiology-directed interventions are carried out by the nursing action. The nurses' activities to change the etiology are documented. The changes, if any, in the etiology component of the nursing diagnosis statement are documented: the client's level of activity (activity theory); the client's level of disengagement (disengagement theory); and the match between the client's preferences and actual activity (continuity theory).

Evaluating

Outcome product evaluation involves evaluating the change in the level of life satisfaction of the client. Nurse-focused outcome process evaluation focuses on the nursing actions actually performed. Client-focused outcome process evaluation focuses on the documented change in the etiology (activity level, disengagement level, or the match between preferences and actual activity).

Colic in the New Born

Infant colic is one of the most common problems encountered in the first year of life (Keefe, 1988). Colic is characterized by paroxysmal abdominal pain and is manifested by loud crying and drawing the legs up toward the abdomen. Colic usually occurs after 3 weeks of age and occurs until approximately 3 months of age. Despite the symptoms the child tolerates feeding well, gains weight, and thrives.

Infant colic is frequently very disturbing to the child and parents. Nurses are often asked to assist a family whose infant is experiencing colic. Four theories, summarized by Keefe (1988), will be illustrated here: the gastrointestinal (GI) theory, the allergy theory, the parental anxiety/tension theory, and the central nervous system (CNS) theory (Table 11.4). Because these theories cite different etiologies for the same phenomena—infant colic—the nursing diagnoses generated from these theories are different and the nursing interventions designed to treat the diagnoses are different.

Assessing

The characteristics of colic provide the structure for assessing. Each theory provides a different focus and structure for assessing the etiology. In the GI

Table 11.4 Summary of Theories of Infant Colic

Phenomena	Characteristics
Colic	Paroxysmal abdominal pain or cramping manifested by loud crying and drawing the legs up to the abdomen. Usually occurs after 3 weeks of age and until approximately 3 months of age. Popularly termed "90-day colic." Despite the obvious behavior indicators of pain, the child tolerates feeding well, gains weight, and thrives.

Theory	Relational Statements
GI Etiology	Infant born with immature GI tract that is ineffective in the peristalic propulsion and expulsion of intestinal gas. GI tract becomes overdistended, resulting in kinking and temporary obstruction. Infant in pain cries which, in turn, results in more swallowed air and pain.
Allergenic Etiology	Pain seen as symptom of an allergy to dietary intake.
Parental Anxiety/Tension Etiology	Child has unsatisfied needs or is overstimulated.
Immature CNS Etiology	Infant has abnormally sensitive CNS; minimal stimuli leads to fussiness and irritability.

theory, the infant is assessed for intestinal gas, swallowed air, and abdominal distention. In the allergy theory, the type of feeding used is assessed; that is, the type of infant formula or foods eaten by the breast-feeding mother. In the parental anxiety/tension theory, the level of anxiety/tension in the parents is assessed. In the CNS theory, the level of environmental stimuli is assessed.

Diagnosing

The major relational statements from each theory are used to generated theory-specific diagnoses (Table 11.4). From the GI etiology theory, the diagnosis could be "colic related to intestinal gas, swallowed air, and abdominal distention." This diagnosis is generated from the relational statements that the GI tract is distended with gas so when the infant cries, more air is swallowed and causes additional abdominal distention. From the allergy etiology theory, the diagnosis could be "colic related to allergy to type of dietary intake." This diagnosis is generated from the relational statement that colic is a symptom of an allergy to dietary intake. From the parental anxiety/tension theory, the diagnose could be "colic related to overly anxious and tense parents." This diagnosis is generated from the relational statement that the child has unsatisfied needs due to overly anxious and tense parents. From the immature CNS theory, the diagnosis could be "colic related to infant's sensitivity to environmental stimuli." This diagnosis is generated from the relational statement that minimal environmental stimuli leads to fussiness and irritability.

Planning

Goals and predicted outcomes are generated from the response component of the diagnosis—infant colic. Resolution of the diagnosis would reflect a decrease in the infant's colic behavior. Interventions are generated from the theory-based etiology components of the diagnoses. Thus, the interventions from the four theories are different.

In the GI etiology theory, efforts are directed at decreasing gas and the swallowing of air in order to decrease abdominal distention. Nursing actions might include burping the infant frequently, using a naturally shaped nipple, and placing the infant in an upright position after feeding.

In the allergy etiology theory, efforts are directed at eliminating the allergy-producing food. Nursing actions might include suggesting a change in formula and/or modifying the breast-feeding mother's diet for foods often associated with allergy.

In the parental anxiety/tension theory, interventions are directed at decreasing the parent's anxiety and tension. Nursing actions might include encouraging the parents to relax and to spend some time away from the infant.

In the CNS theory, interventions are directed at decreasing the environmental stimuli. Nursing actions might include swaddling the infant or leaving the crying infant in the crib for a short time.

Implementing

The etiology-directed interventions are carried out by the nursing actions. the nurses' activities to change the etiology are documented. The changes, if any, in the etiology component of the nursing diagnosis statement are documented: abdominal distention, change to nonallergy producing food, parental anxiety and tension, or the level of stimuli in the environment.

Evaluating

Outcome product evaluation evaluates the change in the infant's colic behavior. Nurse-focused outcome-process evaluation focuses on the nursing actions actually performed. Client focused outcome process evaluation focuses on the documented change in the etiology (abdominal distention, dietary intake, parental anxiety/tension, or level of environmental stimuli).

SUMMARY

This chapter presents a strategy for theory-directed nursing practice. The content of this chapter was used by the authors in developing the demonstration chapters. Descriptions of additional theories utilized by nurses need to be developed and readers are encouraged to try their hand in generating and testing this knowledge for nursing.

REFERENCES

Bloom. M. (1975). *The paradox of helping: Introduction to the philosophy of scientific practice*. New York: John Wiley & Sons.

Burbank, P. M. (1986). Psychosocial theories of aging: A critical evaluation. *Advances in Nursing Science, 9*(1), 73–86.

Burns, N., & Grove, S. K. (1987). *The practice of nursing research: Conduct, critique, and utilization*. Philadelphia: W. B. Saunders.

Fawcett, J., & Downs, F. S. (1986). *The relationship of theory and research*. Norwalk, CT: Appleton-Century-Crofts.

Jacox, A. (1992). Theory construction in nursing—An overview. In L. H. Nicholl (Ed.) *Perspectives on nursing theory* (2nd ed.) (pp. 348–361). Boston: Little, Brown.

Keefe, M. R. (1988). Irritable infant syndrome: Theoretical perspectives and practice implications. *Advances in Nursing Science, 10*(3), 70–78.

Kerlinger, F. N. (1973). *Foundations of behavioral research*, (2nd ed.). New York: Holt, Rinehart & Winston.

La Monica, E. (1990). *Management in nursing: An experiential approach that makes theory work for you.* New York: Springer Publishing Co.

Miller, E. (1989). *How to make nursing diagnosis work: Administrative and clinical strategies.* East Norwalk, CT: Appleton and Lange.

TNA Professional Services Committee (1983). *Problem-solving: A guide for finding solutions.* Pamphlet No. 1 of a series on nurse employment relations. Texas Nurses' Association.

Walker, L. O., & Avant, K. C. (1988). *Strategies for theory construction in nursing.* (2nd ed.) Norwalk, CT: Appleton-Century-Crofts.

Wooldridge, P. J., Leonard, R. C., & Skipper, J. K. (1983). Defining the theory of a practice profession. In P. J. Wooldridge, M. H. Schmitt, J. K. Skipper, and R. C. Leonard. *Behavioral science and nursing theory.* (pp. 1–36). St. Louis: C. V. Mosby.

Zetterberg, H. L. (1965). *On theory and verification in sociology.* (3rd ed.). Totowa, NJ: Bedminster Press.

Ziegler, S. M., Vaughan-Wrobel, B. C., & Erlen, J. A. (1986) *Nursing process, nursing diagnosis, and nursing knowledge: Avenues to autonomy.* Norwalk, CT: Appleton-Century-Crofts.

Appendices

/

APPENDIX A:
GLOSSARY OF NURSING PROCESS TERMS

The terms used in the Nursing Process Model are defined under the step of the nursing process to which they refer.

Assessing

ASSESSING—The process of systematically collecting and organizing information about the client. The process is theory-directed. Information is collected because the theory specifies that particular observations are relevant for understanding the phenomenon of nursing interest.

ASSESSMENT—The product of assessing. The information collected about the client during assessing is documented. This product may be referred to as the client data.

   Subjective Data—Information that the client actually tells the nurse during nursing assessment. Represents the individual, family, group, or community views of self, health, patterns of daily living, demands that are made on them, resources, values, and goals. In the subjective data realm the client is the expert.

   Objective Data—Information obtained by the nurse's (or other health team member's) eye (observation), felt with the hand (palpation/percussion), heard with the ear (ausculation), tasted, or smelled. The nurse describes the observations without drawing conclusions or making interpretations. In the objective data realm the nurse is the expert.

Diagnosing

DIAGNOSING—The process of arriving at a judgment about a client's need for nursing care, based on the data obtained during assessing and documented in the nursing assessment.

DIAGNOSIS—The product of diagnosing. A two-part statement consisting of the actual unhealthful or potential unhealthful client response and the hypothesized cause of the response which is amenable to nursing's independent nursing intervention.

Client Response (actual)—The behavior of the client which is observed by the nurse, compared against theoretical norms, and judged unhealthful.

Client Response (potential)—A prediction of the nurse that certain risk factors are present and that theory predicts will be associated with unhealthful responses in the future.

Etiology—The hypothesized cause of the client's actual or potential unhealthful response, which is amenable to nursing's independent actions. Causation is recognized as multiple in nature. The cause included in the etiology is one that nursing has direct control over and one which is theoretically and/or empirically believed to be a major causative factor. Modification in the etiology is expected to result in a change in the client's response.

Planning

PLANNING—The process of determining the plan for meeting the client's need for nursing care.

NURSING CARE PLAN—The product of care planning. The plan of care is directed by the nursing diagnosis. It includes the client goal(s), predicted outcome(s), nursing intervention(s), and nursing action(s) necessary to individualize nursing care.

Client Goal(s)—The desired client responses stated in the direction of health. Goals are directed by the response component of the nursing diagnosis statement and are highly abstract and standard. They are individualized to the particular client in the client predicted outcomes.

Client Predicted Outcome(s)—The time-specific and measurable client responses the nurse expects to observe after nursing interventions and actions have been implemented. They are individualized to the client. They are generated from standard goals but are unique to the client.

Nursing Intervention(s)—Nursing acts that prevent, modify, remove, or control the factors causing the client's potential or actual unhealthful response. Nursing interventions are etiology-directed and are the means to achieve the client goal(s) and predicted outcomes. They are highly abstract and standard and are individualized to the client in the nursing actions.
Nursing Action(s)—The time-specific and measurable activities planned by the nurse to implement the nursing intervention(s). These are individualized to the client and are generated from standard interventions but are unique to the client.

Implementing

IMPLEMENTING—The process of executing or carrying out the planned nursing actions.
IMPLEMENTATION—The product of implementing. The documentation of the completed nursing actions.

Evaluating

EVALUATING—The process of determining the quality of nursing care.
EVALUATION—The product of evaluating. The documentation of the nurse's actions, the client's actions, and the client's outcomes.
Outcome Product Evaluation—Involves making a judgment about the degree to which the client goal(s) have been achieved. The actual client outcome(s) are compared to the predicted client outcome(s). The judgment is documented and this documentation forms the basis of nursing accountability for the quality of nursing care.
Outcome Process Evaluation—Both the nurse and the client are the focus.
Nurse Focus—Involves making a judgment regarding the extent that nurses carried out the planned nursing actions as evidenced in the documentation. Generated from a comparison of the planned nursing actions and the documented activities of the nurse.
Client Focus—Involves making a judgment regarding the extent that planned nursing actions have been successful in modifying the etiology. Generated from a comparison of the etiology component before and after nursing actions are documented.

APPENDIX B:
GLOSSARY OF THEORY TERMS

Building Blocks of Theory

Concept—"Ideas about classes of ideas derived from experience and expressed through symbols" (Bloom, 1975, p. 37).

Construct—"Constructs are concepts produced by inferences rather than by observations of concrete events" (Bloom, 1975, p. 42).

Variable—The empirical characteristics of concepts that can take on different degrees (Bloom, 1975, p. 43).

Empirical Indicator—"Concepts are not measured directly, but are associated with the empirical indicators explicitly defined as representing those concepts" (Bloom, 1975, p. 43).

Empirical Referent—Same as empirical indicators. "Classes or categories of actual events which by their existence or presence demonstrate the occurrence of the concept" (Walker & Avant, 1988, p. 43).

Sets of Building Blocks of Theory

Proposition—"When two or more concepts are joined together (related), they are wed; they have become a proposition" (Bloom, 1975, p. 44).

Statement—Some authors use the term statement to indicate a proposition (Reynolds, 1971).

Assumptions—Relationships among concepts are assumed true "for purposes of developing a further line of reasoning" (Bloom, 1975, p. 45).

Hypothesis—Relationships among concepts are tested.

Empirical Generalization—Some relationships among concepts are known (have been observed empirically).

Law—"A law states an empirical regularity among phenomena that, as far as is known, is invariable under the conditions of the law" (Jacox, 1992, p. 353).

Any given proposition/statement may be interpreted as falling into any one of the classes (assumption, hypothesis, empirical generalization, law). One person's assumption is another person's hypothesis to be tested, while it is a third person's certain knowledge. One person's empirical generalization is another person's law.

Types of Propositions/Statements

Definitional Proposition/Statement—A statement used to define a concept.
Existence Proposition/Statement—Statements indicating that something exists or is the case.
Relational Proposition/Statement—Statements indicating either an association (correlation) or a causal relationship between concepts.

Set of Propositional Statements

Theory—Network of interrelated propositions/statements (made up of related concepts) which describes, explains, predicts, and provides a sense of understanding of clinical phenomena.

It is relational propositions/statements which provide the basis of prediction and explanation of clinical phenomena.

APPENDIX C:
RATIONALE FOR THE LEVEL OF THEORY
AND SPECIFIC THEORIES SELECTED

The work in nursing concerning the development of a body of nursing knowledge was classified by Walker and Avant (1988) into four levels: meta-theory, grand nursing theory, middle-range theory, and practice theory. Meta-theory focuses on philosophical and methodological questions and is beyond the scope of this book. The other levels of theory are defined and their relevance to the strategy for theory-based nursing practice, as presented in this book, is described.

Grand Nursing Theory (Conceptual Model)

Grand nursing theories "consist of global conceptual frameworks defining broad perspectives for practice and ways of looking at nursing phenomena based on these perspectives" (Walker & Avant, 1988, p. 4). Grand theories, which others would label conceptual nursing models, offer "some general perspectives for practice or curriculum organization in nursing, but by their very nature and purpose most of them would require major revision and expansion before testing would be possible" (Walker & Avant, 1988, p. 9). The concepts and propositions of the conceptual nursing models are highly abstract. Fawcett (1989) stated that "conceptual models are only general guides that must be specified further by relevant and logically congruent theories before action can occur" (p. 26). Thus she claims that conceptual models are not directly applicable in clinical practice.

There are at least seven well-known conceptual nursing models (Fawcett, 1989). Fitzpatrick and Whall (1989) present 23 conceptual models in the second edition of their book. Each of these models presents a different image of the four paradigm concepts of nursing: person, environment, health, and nursing. The models use different concepts and direct the nurse to perceive some phenomena as relevant and other phenomena as not relevant.

Kristjanson, Tamblyn, and Kuypers (1987) identified problems that arise from the application of only one conceptual nursing model to clinical practice. They argued that if perception is limited to only those phenomena which are congruent with a particular model, then recognition of dissonant phenomena in a situation is limited. They asserted that no evidence exists for the assumptions that nursing practice differs under different conceptual frameworks or that improved practice is associated with the adoption of a nursing conceptual model. Lastly, they argued that nurses in practice employ a diversity of theoretical frameworks for practice and use of one conceptual model might inhibit the use of diverse theoretical frameworks.

Thus, the extent to which conceptual nursing models should be used to guide nursing practice remains an issue in the nursing literature. Two diverse points of view were presented by Fitzpatrick and Whall (1984). Fitzpatrick argued that psychiatric nursing practice should be guided by conceptual nursing models. Whall, on the other hand, argued that "harkening back to the authorities of the nursing models may hamper the development of a body of practice-based theory" (p. 47).

Efforts to link conceptual nursing models in nursing research have been evaluated by Silva (1986, 1987). Of the 62 articles she evaluated that focused on tests of five nursing models, 24 made minimal use of the model. She concluded that there was a lack of evidence to show how conceptual nursing models, used as frameworks for research, influence nursing practice.

Diers (1984) and Tripp-Reimer (1984) critiqued two studies presented in the *Western Journal of Nursing Research*. Diers claimed the models appeared extraneous both to the design of the studies and to the eventual conclusions. She concluded "that the research could have been done precisely the same way with precisely the same conclusions and implications without any reference at all to the overhanging models" (p. 191).

Tripp-Reimer (1984) critiqued the same studies. She asserted that using models of nursing as conceptual frameworks for nursing practice research does not advance nursing science. She questioned the value of using nursing conceptual models with studies concerned with interventions.

Middle-Range Theory

Theories of the middle-range are narrower in scope than conceptual models (grand theories), and the concepts and propositions of middle-range theories are less abstract. Middle-range theories fill the gap between conceptual models and nursing practice (Walker & Avant, 1988). Middle-range theories serve to describe, explain, and predict phenomena in the real world. Because they serve these aims of science, they can be used to guide the steps of the nursing process and the problem-solving process.

Middle-range theories are produced by many disciplines. Nursing, as an applied science, has traditionally used the middle-range theories of other disciplines to describe, explain, and predict events in nursing settings. There are no clear guidelines yet established for selecting theories generated in other disciplines for application in nursing.

Nursing Practice

The term practice theory has been widely used in nursing. Walker and Avant (1988) describe practice theory as a practice-oriented level of theory, in which "prescriptions, or more broadly, modalities for practice are delineated" (p. 5). They, as well as Beckstrand (1978), suggested that the use of the term "practice theory" is erroneous. They argued that the essence of practice theory is a desired goal and prescriptions for action to achieve the goal. To Walker and Avant, this represents a "generous extension of the usual meaning of theory" (1988, p. 11). They suggested that the term "practice theory" be dropped and the term "nursing" practices be used instead.

Rationale For Selecting Middle-Range Theory

Middle-range theories are used rather than conceptual nursing models to guide theory-based nursing practice described in this book. Jacox (1992) and Walker and Avant (1988) claimed that propositions most relevant to practice are likely to come from middle-range theories. Because the concepts and propositions of middle-range theories are sufficiently concrete to be useful in describing, explaining, and predicting aspects of nursing practice (Fawcett, 1989), they have been selected to demonstrate the proposed strategy for theory-directed nursing practice, rather than the conceptual nursing models.

SUMMARY

The rationale for the selection of the level and specific theories used to demonstrate theory-based nursing practice in this book is summarized in the following statements.

1. Middle-range theories rather than conceptual nursing models are used. This choice was made because the concepts and propositions of middle-range theories are useful in describing, explaining, and predicting each step of the methodologies of nursing practice—problem solving and nursing process.
2. Theories that nurses in practice believe are useful in guiding practice have been selected for application in the case situations discussed in this book. Nursing as an applied science uses theories developed in other disciplines as well as theories developed by nurses.

REFERENCES

Beckstrand, J. (1978). The need for a practice theory as indicated by the knowledge used in the conduct of practice. *Research in Nursing and Health, 1*, 175–179.

Bloom, M. (1975). *The paradox of helping: Introduction to the philosophy of scientific practice*. New York: John Wiley and Sons.

Diers, D. (1984). Nursing models as conceptual frameworks for research. Commentaries. *Western Journal of Nursing Research, 6*, 191–192.

Fawcett, J. (1989). *Analysis and evaluation of conceptual models of nursing* (2nd ed). Philadelphia: F. A. Davis.

Fitzpatrick, J. J., & Whall, A. L. (1984). Points of View: Should nursing models be used in psychiatric nursing practice. *Journal of Psychosocial Nursing, 6,* 46–47.

Fitzpatrick, J. J., & Whall, A. L. (1989). *Conceptual models of nursing: Analysis and application* (2nd ed.) Norwalk, CT: Appleton & Lange.

Jacox, A. (1992). Theory construction in nursing—An overview. In L. H. Nicholl (Ed.) *Perspectives on nursing theory.* (2nd ed.) (pp. 319–334). Boston: Little, Brown.

Kristjanson, L. J., Tamblyn, R., and Kuypers, J. A. (1987). A model to guide development and application of multiple nursing theories. *Journal of Advanced Nursing, 12,* 523–529.

Reynolds, B. D. (1971). *A primer in theory construction.* Indianapolis: Bobbs-Merrill.

Silva, M. C. (1986). Research testing nursing theory: State of the art. *Advances in Nursing Science, 9,* 1–11.

Silva, M. C. (1987). Conceptual models of nursing. In J. J. Fitzpatrick & R. L. Taunton (Eds.) *Annual review of nursing research* (Vol 5) (pp. 229–246). New York: Springer Publishing Co.

Tripp-Reimer, T. (1984). Nursing models as conceptual frameworks for research. Commentaries. *Western Journal of Nursing Research, 6,* 195–196.

Walker, L. O., & Avant, K. C. (1988). *Strategies for theory construction in nursing* (2nd. ed.). Norwalk, CT: Appleton & Lange.

Author Index

255

Subject Index

⑤ *Springer Publishing Company*

INTERPERSONAL THEORY IN NURSING PRACTICE

Selected Works of Hildegard E. Peplau

Anita W. O'Toole, RN, CS, PhD,
and **Sheila R. Welt**, RN, MS, Editors

*"[Peplau] is a leader who inspires commitment and empowers people
by sharing authority. The editors are to be congratulated for making
Peplau's significant unpublished papers available to all."*
— **Faye G. Abdellah,** *Military Medicine*

*"This book is a gem! Peplau's grounding in the clinical phenomena of
psychiatric nursing and her farsighted vision make these works
eminently useful and stimulating at all levels."* —Nursing Outlook

Translated into Japanese

400pp 0-8261-6060-3 hardcover

EFFECTIVE APPROACHES TO PATIENTS' BEHAVIOR

4th Edition

Gladys B. Lipkin, RNC, MS, CS, FAAN
and **Roberta G. Cohen,** RN, MS, CS

*"The authors make a valuable contribution to nursing literature with
this concise, basic handbook, which will be a useful reference for
nursing students and professionals."*
—American Journal of Nursing
(from a review of the Third Edition)

New to this edition is key coverage of health workers and
personal crisis, homebound patients, patients with chronic or
incurable illness, and crisis intervention.

Nurse's Book Society Selection
Translated into Spanish, Japanese, Dutch, and Portuguese

312pp 0-8261-1496-2 softcover

536 Broadway, New York, NY 10012-3955 • (212) 431-4370 • Fax (212) 941-7842